# YOGA
## *for Movement Disorders*

## Rebuilding Strength, Balance and Flexibility for Parkinson's Disease and Dystonia

# Renée Le Verrier, BS, RYT

Certified Yoga Instructor and Parkinson's disease patient

## Foreword: Lewis Sudarsky, MD

Director, Movement Disorders Clinic, Brigham and Women's Hospital
Associate Professor of Neurology, Harvard Medical School

**Caution:** As with any exercise program, check first with your doctor before practicing the poses presented here. Better yet, show your doctor this book so that he or she can see specifically what you'd like to do. There are precautions for osteoporosis, hip replacement, high blood pressure, glaucoma, as well as other conditions. Your doctor can advise you.

### Author's acknowledgement.
Thank you to the teachers and students I have worked with; I learn from each of you. Very special thanks to Anne Broyles, Diane Davis, dear friend and yoga partner Virginia DePasqua, and, without a doubt, Andreas Meyer. Namaste.

Photographs by Andrew Edgar

Design & Artwork by

**SMK** Design

merit
PUBLISHING
INTERNATIONAL

# YOGA
# *for Movement Disorders*

## Rebuilding Strength, Balance and Flexibility for Parkinson's Disease and Dystonia

**ISBN 978-1-873413-53-1**

**MERIT PUBLISHING INTERNATIONAL**

North American address:
1095 Jupiter Park Drive, Suite 7
Jupiter, FL 33458
USA
Tel: (1) 561 697 1447
Email: meritpi@aol.com

European address:
50 Highpoint, Heath Road
Weybridge, Surrey KT13 8TP
England
Tel: (44) (0) 1932 844526
Email: merituk@aol.com

**www.meritpublishing.com**

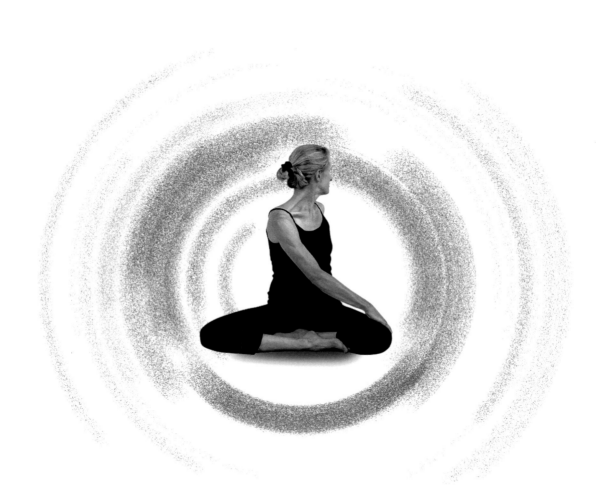

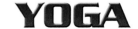
# Contents

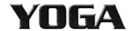

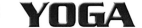

# Foreword

Patients with a neurologic disease can regain some of the mobility they have lost through an exercise program. Le Verrier has put together an instructional guide to yoga with neurologic patients in mind. It is a clear, illustrated text which also touches on her personal journey. Yoga can be the cornerstone of a rehabilitation program for patients with Parkinson's disease, dystonia, and other movement disorders. These exercises also benefit patients with other neurologic problems. This is a graduated approach, but check with your doctor before you embark to ensure that these exercises are appropriate for you.

If you have Parkinson's disease, it's not your fault. We don't presently know the cause or causes of this complex disorder. It is generally considered to be due to a variety of genetic and environmental factors. There is, however, a great deal you can do to optimize your function and minimize the disability related to this disease. These exercises provide benefits to patients with movement disorders which help restore function and complement the effects of medication. Exercise is often as important as medication in getting back some of the motor control that Parkinson's disease has compromised.

People have different goals in mind beginning an exercise program. Some people exercise to improve muscle strength. Some people seek to improve endurance, to expand the capacity of the heart and lungs. These exercises work on flexibility and postural control, which are particular problems for patients with Parkinson's disease and dystonia. Yoga is good for the body as well as the spirit. With practice and teaching, we can all achieve better posture and a more natural manner of movement. When we move through life more effectively, we feel better.

**Lewis Sudarsky, MD**
*Director of Movement Disorders Clinic, Brigham and Women's Hospital*
*Associate Professor of Neurology, Harvard Medical School*

# Preface - Why Yoga?

'[Yoga students] are really happy with who they are.
and they bring a spirit of acceptance – not acceptance
of their limitations. but of who they are in the world [1]'.
– **Peggy Cappy**

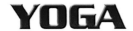

Movement disorders such as Parkinson's disease affect more than the body. They leave a mark on our emotions, sometimes our mental capacity, often our whole spirit.

Tremors, rigidity, and imbalance invade us physically.
As a result, our emotions are held captive. Fear - of falling,
of the progression of the toxin in our brains or that another
blood vessel will burst, of losing so much - takes over
our thoughts. Then, there's struggle. The simplest
movements - the dexterity needed to uncap the toothpaste or hold the spoon steady enough to eat a cup of soup - are monumental challenges that erode our ability to stay positive.

Moving through the poses and flows of yoga helps reduce muscle rigidity and increases strength, balance and flexibility. Yoga also affects more than the body; it balances our emotions, calms our mind, and creates peace in our spirit.

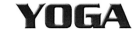

# Part 1

# Introduction

## Chapter 1
## THE PATH HOME

'Just tell the truth to yourself of what it is because what is not acknowledged cannot be healed [2]'.
– Lilias Folan

**THE DIAGNOSIS**

My symptoms confused neurologists at first. They confused and terrified me, too. A force was taking over my body. It was the tiger.

The tiger was my worst fear as a child. I was convinced that one would leap through my bedroom window while I slept. I lay on my bed peering at the curtain. It wasn't the summer breeze that made it flutter, it was tiger's breath. He was out there.

At the end of my eleventh summer, the tiger visited. I recognized him immediately, even though he didn't appear in his traditional black stripes or jump in through the window. He did, however, pounce and leave his mark.

This tiger was in my brain. I'd been born with an AVM – an arteriovenous malformation. A twisted mass of blood vessels, an AVM can linger undetected anywhere in the body until it bursts. I was in the eighth grade when it turned the left half my body to lead. I'd had a stroke.

When I walked out of the month long hospital stay, bald from the surgery, my left leg dragged behind. But with physical therapy, it gained some strength and balance. My right leg kicked in most of the effort and though I was anything but symmetrical, I hiked, I bicycled, I swam.

So, thirty-five years later, when my left leg started getting stiffer, less responsive, I again heard the tiger growl. Did I have another AVM? I also felt my right wrist and fingers lose coordination. Did I have two AVMs?

Neurologist number one diagnosed Parkinson's disease. He explained that the disease causes stiffness all over; affecting weak areas first and that explained the decrease in the use of my left leg. He added that the disease itself was attacking the right arm and leg.

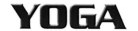 
No, that would be just too cruel, even for a hungry tiger. I'd be out of sides. Parkinson's became a four-letter word. It wasn't spoken aloud in the house. If reference had to be made to it, we didn't say *Parkinson's*. We called it *The P-word*. I sought a second opinion. I sought any opinion that wouldn't pounce and take control over me.

Neurologist number two declared, "Not" The P-word. *Hooray*.

Clinging to number two's *Not*, I went neurologist-free for a year. My symptoms remained. Actually, they got worse. A tremor crept into my thumb. I stumbled.

Neurologist number three said it looked like a mild stroke. I can handle stroke, I thought. Did that, been there. Nice tiger. One recovers from a stroke. I voted for stroke. But symptoms canceled out my vote. I started moving in slow motion, lost my balance while standing at the dryer folding laundry.

Neurologists number four and five concurred: The P-word. My worst fear. The scariest tiger yet. Oh, string of four-letter words.

## MY YOGA JOURNEY

Duane wore baggy sweats with oversized T-shirts. He taught at the Y. When I entered his class for the first time - my first time in any yoga class - he looked as though he'd be as comfortable on the couch with the TV remote as he did on the towel he used as a mat.

I liked that. He didn't seem like he'd wrap his leg around his head in some advanced pose and expect the class to do the same. I really liked that.

I wanted a stretching class. We stretched. But we also breathed and became aware of sensations in our bodies. It was in his class that I first heard "Don't judge. Simply observe." *Don't judge?* Don't harangue my body for losing balance in tree pose? Don't frown for not being able to straighten my legs in down dog?

Duane's statement freed a lot of brain space. I hadn't realized all the chatter going on up there. With his words *don't judge*, clouds floated away. If entering the Y's fitness room was my first step toward yoga, *don't judge* was the long jump toward something bigger than just stretching. He had me connecting with my body, listening to what it said. By clearing the monologue in my head, I could hear so much more.

I was learning to rest comfortably in the present, instead of worrying about the past or fretting about the future. Any body, I discovered, even one with Parkinson's, can find that calm abiding place. When I'm there, I'm not saddened by loss because the past is truly behind me. When I'm there, I'm not afraid because my fears are *what ifs* of the future. When I'm there, I'm truly here.

Teaching and practicing yoga has given me strength. My arms, legs, core abdominal muscles all carry me straighter and with more ease. I've

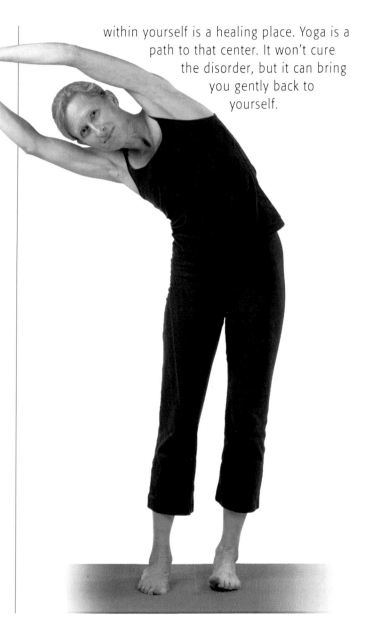

discovered my balance has improved. And even when my medication dose wanes, I'm not as rigid. The inner strength and balance I've gained has also led me to witness what is and accept it. At times, even embrace it. I'm becoming as comfortable in my body as Duane looked in his that first day in class.

## THE PROGNOSIS

I say it aloud now. *"Parkinson's"*. I can even put it in the same sentence with "I" and "have." But it doesn't have me. It is through yoga - its poses, self-reflection, living in the present - that I've learned to no longer fear the tiger. Oh, it's still here. But it doesn't pounce or take control anymore. I've tamed him and we live side by side.

## YOUR YOGA JOURNEY

Living with a movement disorder is a challenge. The array of symptoms and the prognosis for cures can bring fear, struggle and loss of spirit, derailing our emotions, relationships, life as it was. In addition, the physical hurdles - stiffness, facial tics, rigidity, loss of balance, weakness, awkward movements - are there every day, every moment.

Whatever led to your diagnosis and wherever you are in living with your symptoms, practicing yoga can help you get back in balance emotionally and physically. The non-judgmental, peaceful center within yourself is a healing place. Yoga is a path to that center. It won't cure the disorder, but it can bring you gently back to yourself.

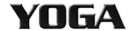
# Chapter 2
# BEFORE YOU BEGIN

'Wisely and slow. They stumble that run fast'.
– Romeo and Juliet, William Shakespeare

In yoga practice, certain poses prepare us for other poses. Mind and body connect and breath, movement, and a gradual turning inward all support one another.

It's like a crossword puzzle. The challenge is to find the working combination of letters to fit together across and down, playing off each other, one word supporting another.

## BEGINNING YOUR PRACTICE

Each day as the week progresses, the *New York Times* crossword puzzles increase in difficulty. Beginners start with Monday's entry, filling in the answers in pencil. Within a couple of weeks, they might even try Tuesday's puzzle.

With practice, veterans get to know the common clues and grow to understand the nuance in others. They switch to using a pen. Over time, they sail through to Friday's grid, building up to the challenge of the weekend puzzles.

This ease-into-it approach is a good way to begin yoga. This holds true particularly with the muscle

rigidity and balance concerns that come with movement disorders. Overworking rigid muscles can cause spasms. Stretching too far can tear soft tissue. Coming into and out of a pose with too much force can cause an injury or a fall. This is gentle yoga where less is more. Be gentle with yourself.

Begin simply. Start with the Warm-ups in Chapter three and practice a few at a time. Get to know them, in your mind and in your body. Add a few more to your practice and then include a few steps from one of the chapter's list of poses, alternating days for variety. If you begin to struggle, take a break.

In yoga, movement follows the breath. Typically, we exhale into a pose and inhale coming out of the pose, allowing the body to flow with the wave of our breathing. The steps for each of the poses note if the movement is done on an inhale or exhale. Most importantly, breathe fully and follow your rhythm of breathing. If your breath is strained, your body is likely to be, too.

A 'difficulty level' description appears below each set of poses in Chapters four through 10. In most chapters,

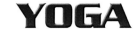

there are seated and standing variations of the same flow. The seated variation works most, if not all, of the same muscle groups as the standing variation, but with the stability of sitting in a chair.

It is helpful to move through the seated option first, even if you're able to try the standing version. This lets your muscles get a sense of the stretches at a base level. Once you're standing, stay near the chair to reach out for the chair back for support at any time. I've found I feel safe using a chair both seated and for support when standing. I can stretch with better alignment and more deeply because I'm not worried about losing my balance.

If you're new to yoga, welcome. If you've practiced yoga before and you're returning to it, welcome back. Take pleasure easing into it.

## WHEN AND WHERE

What is the ideal setting for practicing yoga? Unlike a crossword puzzle where only one answer fits, there are many options for when and where yoga can fit into your day. Select a time that is quiet and the most comfortable space for you and your schedule.

It's a good idea to wait at least an hour after eating before doing any asana, or poses. Many find that early morning practice works best, before breakfast but after the first round of medication. Whatever time you decide, schedule an extra half hour on either side so you're not rushed to begin or end.

An hour is a standard length of a yoga class. Some are forty-five minutes, some up to two hours. The flows in this book vary but on average take an hour. If you have more time, take an extra few minutes at the beginning and end, the opening breathing practice and closing guided imagery. If you have less time, do fewer poses. The Coming to Stillness and Relaxation aspects of the practice are as beneficial as the asana practice.

Select a room that is comfortable and as free from distractions as possible. When you set up your mat and chair, be certain there are no end tables or other obstacles near enough to injure you if you fall. Consider setting up near a wall for an additional place to reach out for balance should you need it. If transferring to a chair is difficult, you can sit on the edge of your bed. Place a folded towel or small pillow under your sitting bones so your hips are level or tilted forward slightly and not curving down into the bed.

Consider personalizing your space with candles, flowers or a memento that is meaningful to you. Each time you step on the mat or sit in the chair, you'll know you're somewhere special.

## WHAT TO WEAR

Clothes that allow you to move and stretch work best for yoga. Opt for elastic or drawstring waistbands rather than snaps and zippers. Avoid buttons in tops as they may dig into your skin in a reclined position. Also, tops that are too loose can both get in the way when twisting and slip over your head when bending forward.

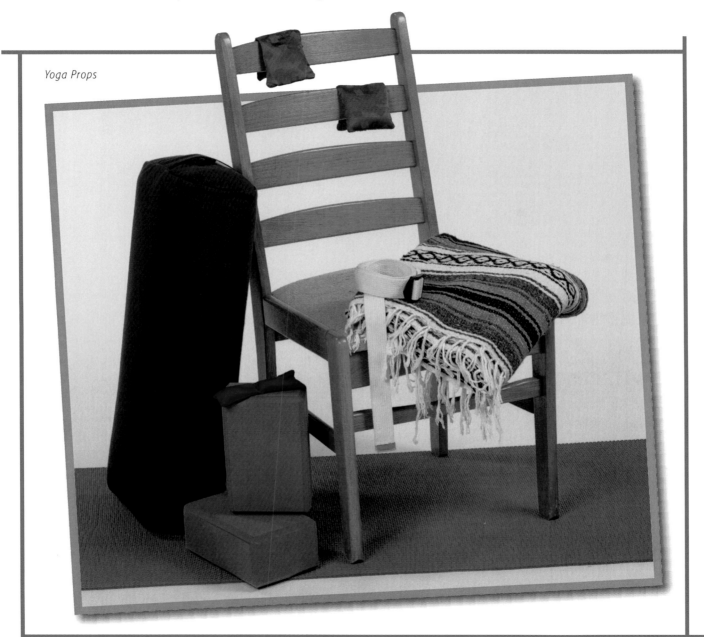

*Yoga Props*

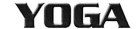
There's no need to purchase special exercise wear. The main reason many yoga teachers and students don yoga or sports clothing is that it is form-fitting. This not only keeps excess fabric out of the way, it allows for observation. When a teacher demonstrates a pose, the students can see the positioning better than if the instructor is wearing a baggy outfit. The same holds true for the teacher being able to see if the student is in a safe position when in a pose, and not, for example, overextending a knee.

Try to practice barefoot. The sensation of the mat on the bottom of our feet helps with balance and you'll get more traction in standing poses, which will prevent injury from slipping. Besides, it gives your toes some freedom.

## PROPS

Movement disorders throw us out of alignment, whether from one-sided weakness, muscle rigidity, slow movement, or spasms. Alignment is an essential factor in yoga. Joints function at their best when lined up properly with good blood flow. Nerves don't get pinched and energy moves. Proper alignment also prevents injury from overstretching or straining areas that don't move freely.

I haven't been symmetrical since the seventh grade. But I can be with props. Props help you straighten where you need it. Sitting on the edge of a cushion, for example, can put your hips in a neutral position, lengthening your back without strain. Light weights

such as sandbags or sacks of rice help calm tremors, allowing an arm to relax instead of curl up with tension.

A chair not only raises the floor closer to your upper body, it provides stability when sitting or standing. Blocks also bring the floor closer so you won't strain your back or hamstrings reaching for the floor. A book or stack of books can substitute for blocks.

Bolsters provide support in reclining positions. Sofa cushions make good bolsters. Straps can be used to support, give added length to your arms when you can't reach. Use a webbed, cloth belt in lieu of a yoga strap.

And the mat itself, often called a 'sticky mat,' prevents slipping. Using props can make the difference between a healthy yoga practice and one fraught with injury.

## CHAPTER FORMAT

Part one prepares you for practicing yoga. Part two presents a daily guide to yoga practice. The chapters flow as a yoga class does, with an initial centering or calming few moments followed by warm-up movements that lead to the poses. The practice ends with relaxation.

There are two additional segments that highlight the particular benefits of the poses and that suggest ways to carry your yoga into the rest of your day.

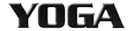 
## ASANA PRACTICE

### Coming to stillness

These few moments allow for the transition from what you were doing before yoga to your practice. The focus is on breath work, which helps bring your focus away from the day's tasks or pondering what's for dinner and back to yourself, in your body, in the present moment.

### Warm-ups

Chapter three details the warm-up poses. Begin with the warm-ups. Don't skip them. They're good for you. They're fat-free, dairy-free, gluten-free, and will help keep you injury-free. Take it slowly. Yoga is a wonderful tool but not a quick fix.

### Poses

The week brings you full circle. Like moving from sunrise to sunset, the full seven days cover calming, strength, balance, flexibility, and relaxation poses.

Each chapter revolves around a theme for that day. Sunday focuses on the sun, with sun salutations. Monday introduces the moon series. Tuesday describes the benefits and how-to-steps of twists while Wednesday covers breathing exercises and why they're so beneficial. Thursday's asana practice works on building strength and balance and Friday pulls it all together in a series of poses that flow from one to the next. Saturday, the traditional day of rest, invites you into restorative poses.

### Relaxation

Yoga classes routinely end with a final pose called *savasana*, which translates as the corpse pose. It is a restful several minutes – preferably twenty but at least ten – where you lie comfortably and let go of thoughts and active movement and allow your body to absorb the benefits of the poses. The longer and deeper the relaxation, the better it is for the body because healing occurs when we are in this state of ease.

Each chapter ends with a guided relaxation to help lead you into the restful pose of savasana. Transitioning into this relaxed pose involves easing down onto the mat and arranging your blankets or bolsters. The Variations section in Chapter three suggests how to get down onto the floor using a chair. If you find it difficult to get down onto the floor, you can raise your legs onto another chair. You can also have your chair positioned near a bed or couch so you can put your feet up.

Take a few minutes to be sure you're comfortable, whether you're on the floor or in a chair. Reposition if you need it so that you'll be comfortable for the full ten to twenty minutes. Consider covering up with a blanket. Our bodies cool down without movement, and it is difficult to fully relax if you get chilled.

It is helpful to have someone read the guided imagery pieces to you. Or, you may want to record yourself reading the guided pieces to play during savasana.

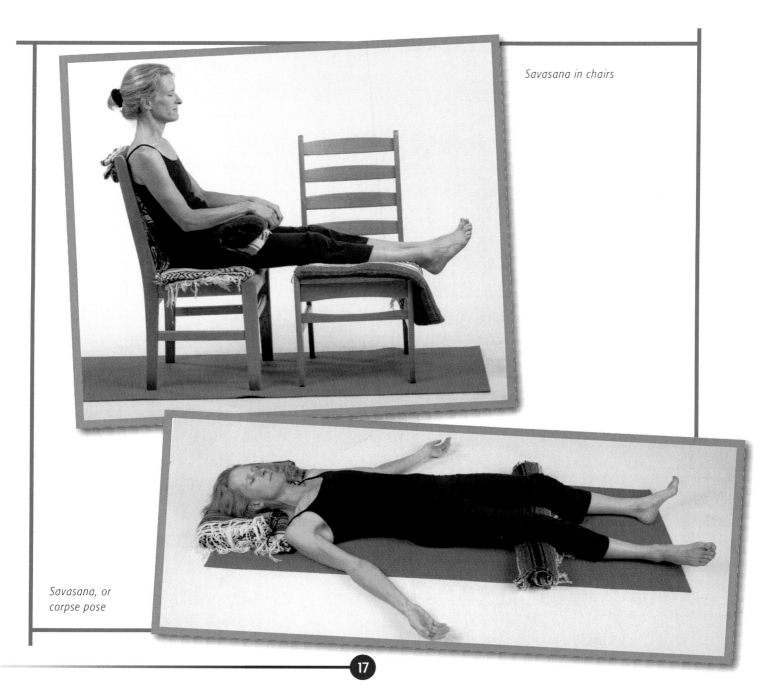

*Savasana in chairs*

*Savasana, or corpse pose*

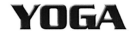
As important as settling into savasana is coming out of it. Take your time coming out of this final pose. Open your eyes slowly. Sit up with care. Let the relaxed state stay with you.

### ESPECIALLY BENEFICIAL

This list follows the asana practice and highlights the aspects of the poses that are of particular help in alleviating symptoms of movement disorders. It mentions muscle groups as well as functionality of a certain area.

### YOGA-TO-GO: APPLYING IT TO YOUR DAY

This final list suggests ways to continue your yoga after you've rolled up the mat. Simply being aware of your breath at times throughout the day brings your mind and body together. These ideas aim at making that connection in everyday living.

# WORDS OF CAUTION

### CHECK WITH YOUR DOCTOR

As with any exercise program, check first with your doctor before practicing the poses presented here. Better yet, show your doctor this book so that he or she can see specifically what you'd like to do. There are precautions for osteoporosis, hip replacement, high blood pressure, glaucoma, as well as other conditions. Your doctor can advise you.

### BE SAFE

If you're not confident about your balance, practice in a chair. Be sure all four legs of the chair are on a sticky mat to prevent sliding. Place your chair away from end tables and anything else that might cause injury if you fall from the chair.

Use the chair for support. Pause at any time you feel you need a rest. Ease up at any time you feel pain. Stop at any time you feel dizzy. Smile any time you feel good.

### TAKE YOUR TIME

Some poses are simple enough to move in and out of with little effort or time. Others need you to take them slowly. All are most beneficial when approached gently and with focus.

Ladder grams are word puzzles that can be deceptively easy. They list a beginning and end word. By changing one letter in the first word once for each of a number of steps, you arrive at the end word. Some are quick games that need only three or four steps. Most are more challenging and take more time and concentration.

Rebuilding strength, flexibility and balance from weak and stiff muscles caused by a neurologically-based disorder can't be done quickly. The poses and exercises in this book will help you move toward strength and flexibility. Like a ladder gram, moving from rigid to fluid will take more than a few simple steps.

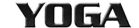

## NOTE TO TEACHERS

### Safety

If you're using chairs in your class and have students with balance concerns, please space the chairs out. Try to keep them ten feet from each other. In case someone does lose their balance, another person is less likely to be affected. Also, be sure that all four legs of the chair are on the mat during practice to prevent slippage.

Some symptoms of movement disorders affect cognition. The first few minutes after a deep relaxation can increase any confusion. If you can, incorporate an additional five or ten minute after savasana for business updates – schedule changes and such – or a discussion or a social time to allow for the transition. This is helpful for those who drove themselves as well as for anyone waiting for a ride. Please make an extra mental note to be sure each student has a way home after class.

### Poses

If you plan to teach the modified poses in this book, practice them yourself and sense the energy of each, the standing and the sitting variations. Know them. Don't simply move into them, feel them. Note how the movement feels in your body.

Remember that it feels different in your students' bodies. While this is true for any yoga instruction, it is particularly so when working with people with movement disorders because nerve connections and pathways work differently. They're blocked or triggers cause involuntary rather than voluntary movement. You can't know what's happening in their bodies. You can, however, as you would with any student, observe and listen. Learn from them and modify these poses as you need for your students.

Flowing in and out of poses is more beneficial to a student with a movement disorder than is holding a pose for any length of time. Holding a pose can trigger involuntary muscle contraction, spasms, and overheating. Move gently and allow for resting breaths, which is a healthy approach on or off the mat.

# Chapter 3
# WARM-UPS

'**Warm:** to infuse with the feeling of love,
friendship, well-being, or pleasure
**up:** in or into a better or more advanced state'.
– **Merriam-Webster's Collegiate Dictionary**

She shuffled in to the hospital cafeteria with a man wearing a staff badge. The two settled into a table next to the picture window. His tag said Physical Therapist after his name, but they didn't appear to be engaged in any exercises. The woman sat straighter than she had stood, her white hair cropped close, her gaze out into the parking lot.

A man walking a brown and white beagle mix appeared on the sidewalk. The woman sat straighter still. The man scooped up the dog and held it to the glass as he smiled and mouthed something inaudible. The woman beamed, pressing her palm on the pane. The dog wagged and wriggled. The man blew her a kiss, waved, and continued down the sidewalk. The woman turned to her therapist and said, "I'm ready now." And she rose and shuffled out of the cafeteria with him.

## ASANA PRACTICE

Warming up prepares us both physically and mentally for the poses we move into afterwards. Loosening up tight spots is only part of the process. We're also quieting our minds and bringing our awareness to our bodies in motion, which means we're less likely to get injured from overstretching, straining, or overheating.

These initial poses also remind us to move with our breath. As you get to know the routine, following the rhythm of your breathing will become natural.

To begin, find a comfortable seated position on a cushion or a straight-backed chair. Work through the Set A of the warm-up poses in order, from the neck down the spine. Notice how your body feels after each one. It may be enough for you physically or time-wise to stop after the set. Or, continue into the poses of any of the daily flows.

Together, the poses in Set A bend, stretch, flex and twist the spine in all the directions it's meant to move. The second set works specific areas. The chapters in Part 2 indicate which pose from Set B to add to your routine for the day's practice. You can also choose one or more on your own to do during any day of your practice.

At any time throughout the warm-ups, if you need to take a break, please do. Pause and take a resting breath.

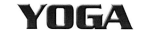
Mentally scan your body from head to toe and notice what's going on – aches, pockets of mobility that weren't previously there, a shift, no shift at all. In following my first teacher, Duane's advice, *Don't judge*. Simply notice.

# SET A

*Needed: Straight-backed chair, Sticky mat*

### 1. SEATED MOUNTAIN

a. This is the base pose for starting any seated position. It is quite active considering it looks as though we're simply sitting in a chair.

b. Sit at the front edge of your chair, your feet about hip width apart on the mat and your weight evenly balanced on both sitting bones, which are located at the center of each buttock.

c. Lengthen your spine by pressing up through the crown of your head, as though you're trying to touch the ceiling with the tassel of an imaginary hat.

d. Create space between your hips and your ribs, reaching upward but keeping your shoulders relaxed.

e. Try to broaden your shoulders. Raise your sternum, or breastbone, up toward the ceiling slightly, and tuck your chin slightly.

f. Let your arms drop to your sides and reach through to your fingertips.

g. And breathe.

h. Return your hands to your thighs or lap.

i. Begin each of the seated warm-ups with this pose.

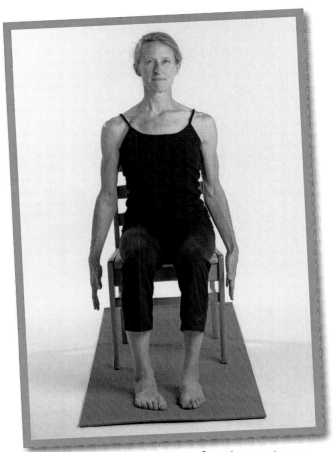

*Seated mountain pose*

## 2. NECK RELEASES

a. These invite joint fluids into the cervical disks and helps release tension.

b. From seated mountain pose, exhale and drop your chin to chest.

c. Inhale. Exhale and turn to look over your right shoulder. Inhale to center and exhale your chin to look over your left shoulder.

d. Move through another cycle of breath. Inhale your head back to center.

e. On an exhale, drop your right ear to your right shoulder. Inhale back up. Exhale and drop your left ear to left shoulder. Inhale back up.

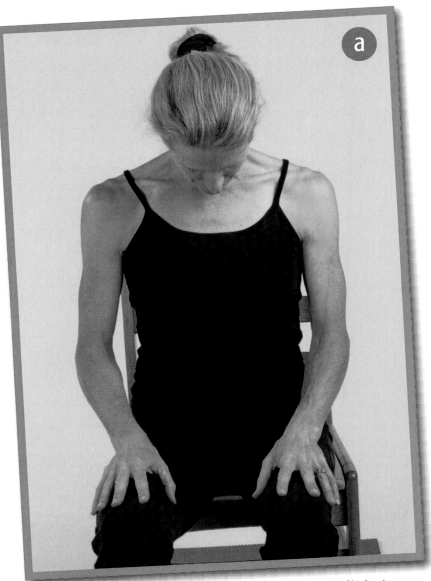

*Neck releases*

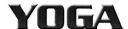

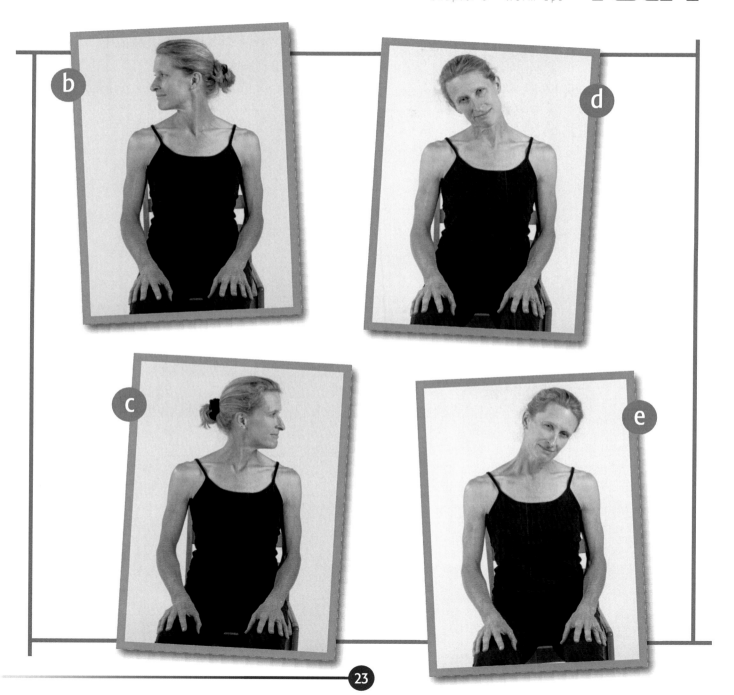

## 3. SHOULDER ROLLS

a.  These unlock some of the many muscles and tendons that make up the shoulder.

b.  Inhale and raise your shoulders up, exhale and circle them back and around and down. Try this three times and reverse direction for three rounds. If more feels better, try a few more.

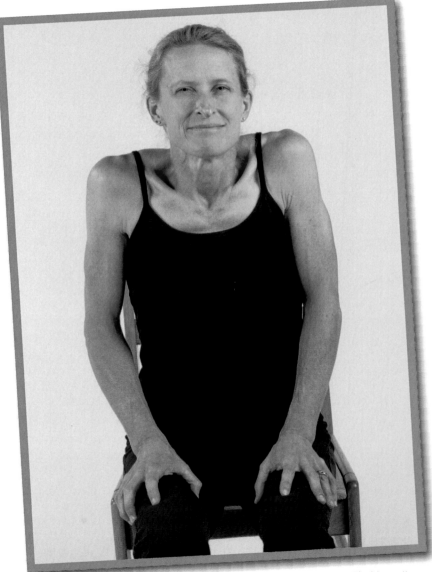

*Sholder rolls*

### 4. WRIST STRETCHES

a.  These coax blood into your fingers and free up some rigidity in the wrists.

b.  Extend your arms in front of you, palms up. Take hold of your right fingertips with your left hand and on an exhale, press them toward the floor. Release and switch hands.

c.  With your arms extended in front of you, turn your palms down. Take hold of your right fingertips with your left hand and on an exhale, press them toward the floor. Release and switch hands.

d.  Release your hands back to your lap.

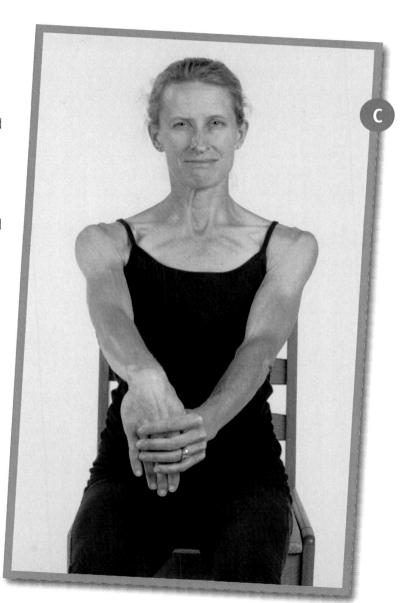

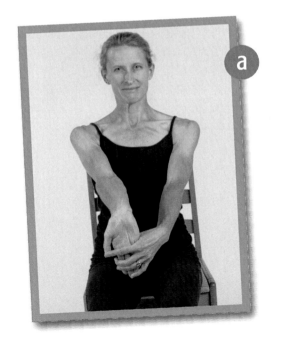

*Wrist stretches*

## 5. UPWARD SALUTE

a.  This asana stretches the intercostals, the muscles between the ribs, opening up our breathing area. It is also the beginning pose of a sun salutation, a way of greeting the day. I often take the opportunity in this pose to welcome what will come in the day, or state an intention I may have for that day, such as *Really listen today* or *Be patient*.

b.  Drop your arms to your sides, palms out.

c.  Inhale and raise your arms to the ceiling with straight elbows and reaching fingertips. If it's comfortable for your neck, look up at your hands.

d.  Turn your palms outward and exhale your arms down, following your fingertips with your gaze.

e.  Repeat two more times.

f.  Note that if one arm is weaker, raise the stronger arm first and try the variation using a strap that follows.

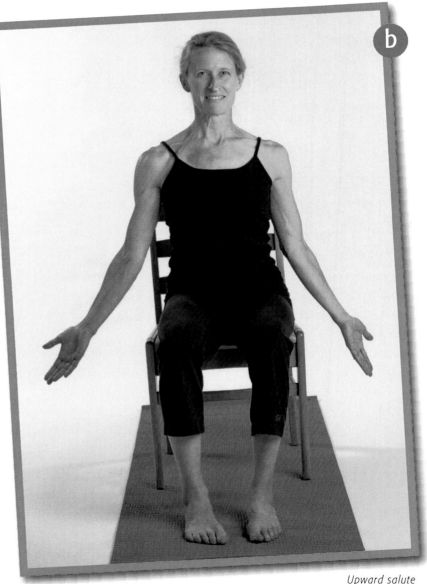

*Upward salute*

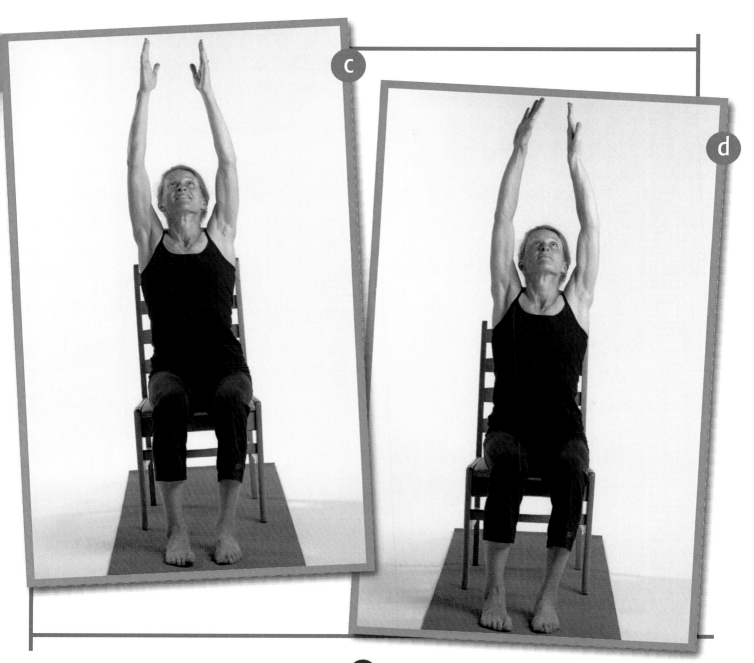

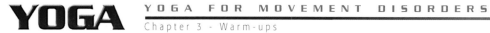

## 6. LATERAL STRETCH

a. This is another stretch for the intercostals as well as the muscles in the hip and shoulder.

b. Drop to your arms to your sides. For support, place your left hand on the chair seat beside your left hip.

c. Inhale and raise your right arm to the ceiling, your upper arm beside your right ear.

d. Exhale and reach the right hand to the left.

e. Inhale your arm to straight overhead and exhale it down to your side.

f. Repeat for the left side.

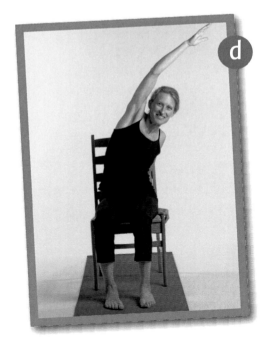

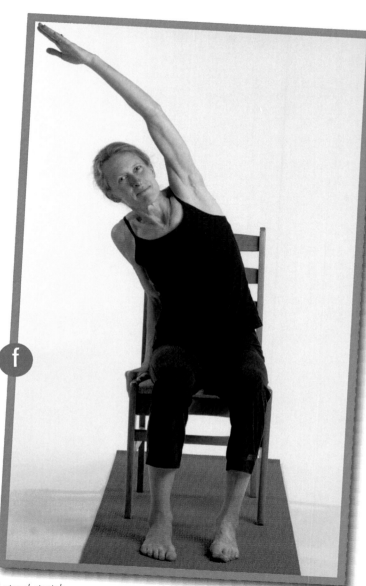

*Lateral stretch*

### 7. CAT AND DOG

a. These flex and extend the vertebrae of the spine, creating space and welcoming in joint fluids.

b. Place your palms on your thighs. Inhale, and with an exhale, press your spine toward the back of the chair, rounding your shoulders forward and dropping your chin.

c. Inhale as you press your spine and navel forward, pressing your sternum up slightly, your shoulders back.

d. For two more cycles of breath, exhale into cat, rounding your spine, and inhale into dog, arching your spine.

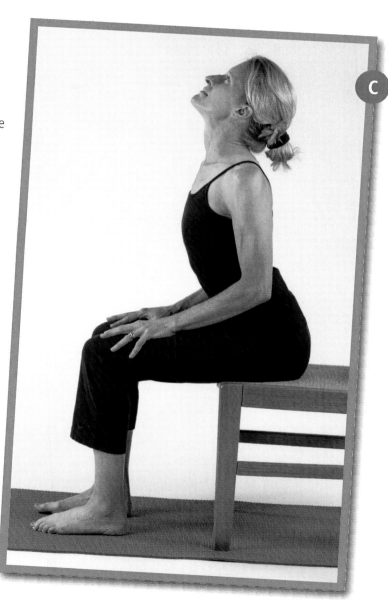

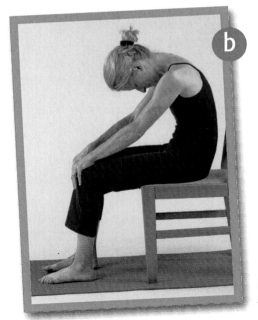

*Cat stretch*

*Dog stretch*

## 8. TWIST

a. Place your left hand on the outside of your right knee. Place your right hand on the chair behind your right hip.

b. Place enough weight onto your right sitting bone to free up your left hip so it can move with the twist.

c. Inhale and lengthen straight up.

d. Exhale and twist your belly to the right.

e. Inhale and lengthen up. Exhale and twist your rib cage to the right.

f. Inhale and lengthen up. Exhale and twist your shoulders to the right. If it's comfortable, look over your right shoulder.

g. Use your arms for extra leverage as needed.

h. Inhale as you gently untwist. Rest your palms on your lap.

i. Repeat on the left side.

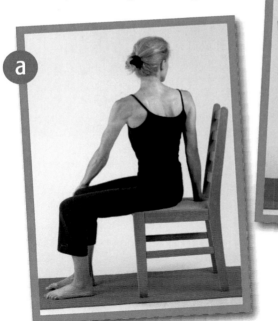

*Twist*

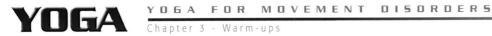

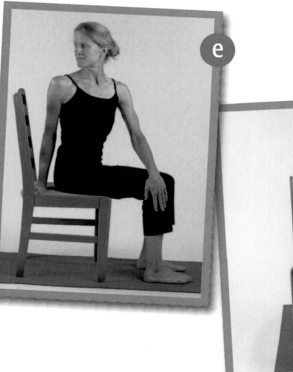

*Twist, front view*

## 9. FORWARD BEND

a. Inhale and on an exhale, hinge forward at the hips keeping a straight back.

b. Reach your palms toward the mat or on blocks beside your feet. Or, keep your palms on your thighs for support, protecting your lower back.

c. Inhale back to center.

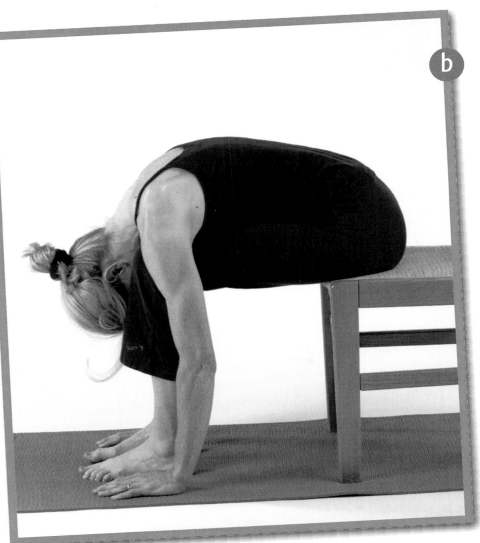

*Forward bend, side view*

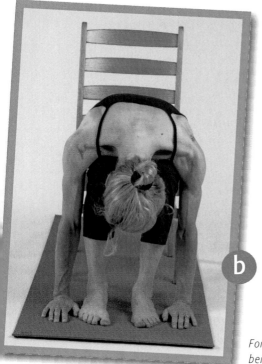

*Forward bend*

*Sholder opener hug*

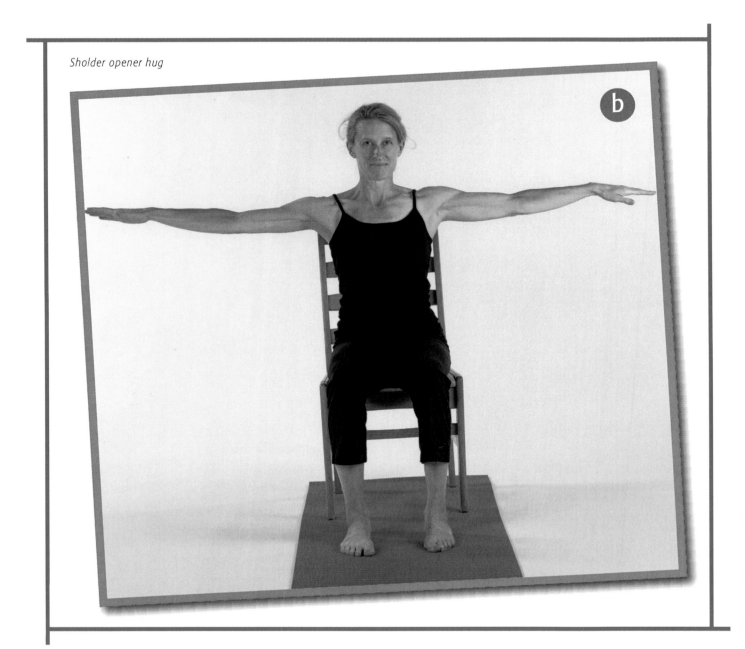

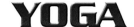
# SET B

## 1. HUG

a. This opens the scapular area, or, the shoulder blades.

b. From seated mountain, extend your arms into a T position, reaching out through your fingertips.

c. Inhale, and on an exhale, bring your arms across your chest and wrap your hands around opposite shoulders. Notice which arm is on top.

d. On an exhale, turn your head to look over your right shoulder. Inhale back to center. Linger in the hug for a moment and note how it feels. On the next exhale, turn your head to look over your left shoulder.

e. Remembering which arm is on top, inhale back to T position and repeat steps c and d with the other arm on top.

f. Release and bring your hands back to your thighs.

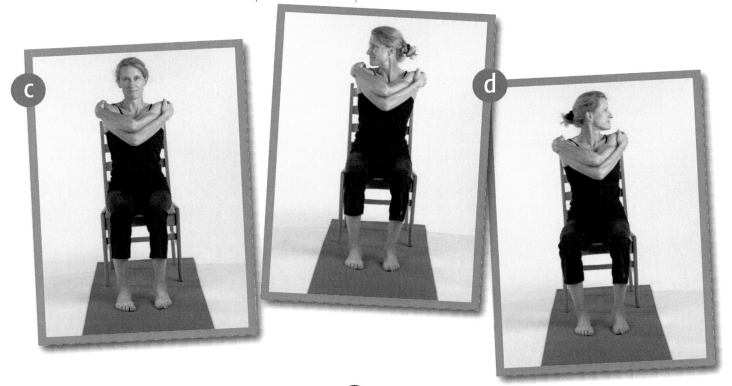

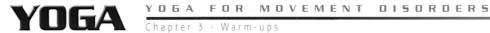

## 2. CIRCLE FROM HIPS

a.  This lower back opener also releases the hips some.

b.  Place your hands on your lap or at your waist.

c.  Hinging at the hips rather than the waist, circle your torso clockwise, following your breath with the movement by exhaling forward and inhaling as you circle your upper body back. Reverse direction.

d.  A way of trying to keep your back straight as you circle, imagine a paintbrush at the top of your head and you're painting big circles on he ceiling.

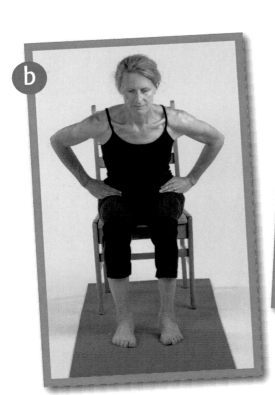

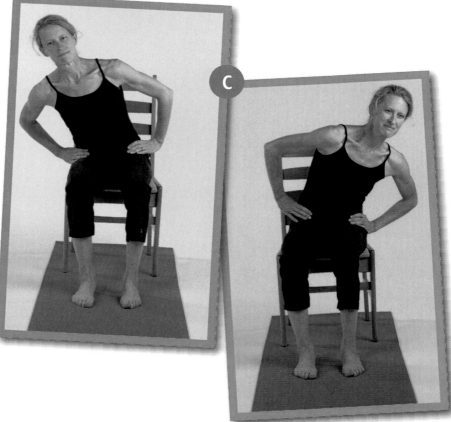

*Hip circle*

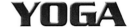
## 3. FOOT STRETCH

a. Oh, the forgotten feet. This stretches the many muscles in the arch and top of the feet, which are so important for balance.

b. Position your feet as if you're standing on tip toes, your foot as close as possible to a right angle to your toes. Hold the position for two rounds of breath.

c. Release and allow the left foot to be flat on the mat. Kick your right foot back, the top of your toes on the mat. Press into you foot slightly and hold the position for two rounds of breath.

d. Repeat for the left foot.

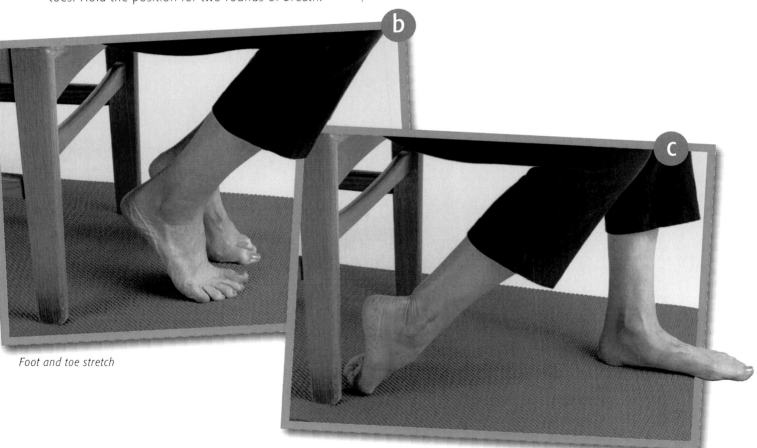

*Foot and toe stretch*

## 4. HEAD TO KNEE

a. This movement works the quadriceps in our front thighs and stretches the hamstrings in the back thighs. The extra bonus is that is also strengthens the abdominals. This is especially beneficial because the core muscles of the stomach and back carry us through when arms and legs are weak.

b. On an inhale, kick the right foot out, straightening that leg. Exhaling, bend your knee up towards your chest, rounding your back and reaching your arms around the bent leg.

c. Following the breath, repeat three more times.

d. Take a moment to notice how each leg feels before repeating with the left leg.

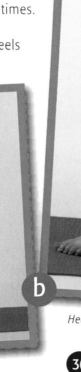

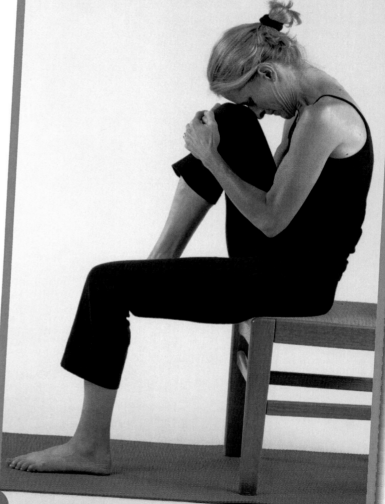

*Head to knee*

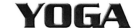

## 5. STANDING TWIST

a. If you're able to stand safely and comfortably, step behind your chair, several inches away. You can reach out for the chair back for support at any time. Be sure that all four legs of the chair are still on the mat.

b. Let your arms hang loosely at your sides. Swing from side to side, allowing your arms to follow the motion like empty coat sleeves.

As your weight shifts onto your right leg, try to lift your left heel off the mat slightly so your left foot pivots a bit and keeps in line with your knee. Do the same with the right.

c. For more balance, hold onto the chair back with your right hand and twist your left arm to the left. As you swing baack to center, switch hands and twist your right arm to the right.

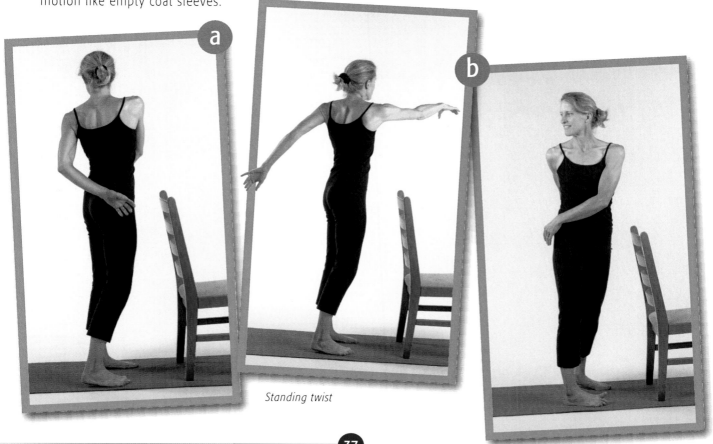

*Standing twist*

## 6. STANDING MOUNTAIN

a. This is the base pose for starting any standing position. It, too, like seated mountain, is an active pose.

b. Stand a few inches behind your chair, your weight evenly balanced on both feet. If you can, spread your toes wide. Feel the bottoms of your feet at the ball of your big toes as well as at the ball of your little toes. Notice the bottom of your heels on the inner as well as the outer edges.

c. Lift your kneecaps up by tightening your thighs. At the same time, try to pull your buttocks muscles down slightly.

d. Lengthen your spine by pressing up through the crown of your head, as though you're trying to touch the ceiling with the tassel of an imaginary hat.

e. Create space between your hips and your ribs, reaching upward but keeping your shoulders relaxed.

f. Try to broaden your shoulders. Raise your sternum, or breastbone, up toward the ceiling slightly, and tuck your chin slightly.

g. Let your arms drop to your sides and reach through to your fingertips.

h. And breathe.

i. Release and smile.

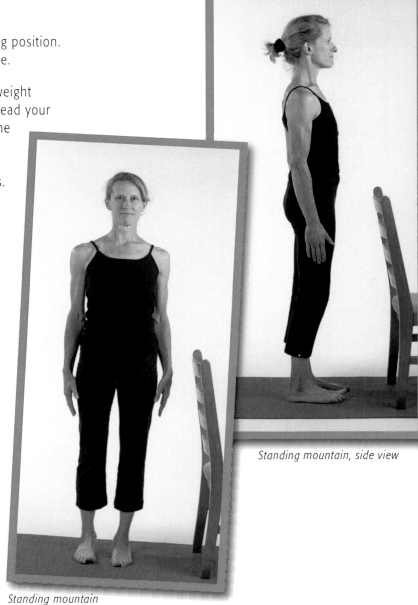

*Standing mountain, side view*

*Standing mountain*

## VARIATIONS

I've often smiled to myself in a yoga class when the teacher asks us to notice how our right side and left side may feel different from one another. May? I can't remember when it felt the same.

With many movement disorders, there's an imbalance, whether it's involuntary stiffness in one leg or an arm that doesn't respond quite as it should or tremors or spasms. Fighting against those movements is not only frustrating; it can make the tension stronger. And, it takes your focus away from your breath, from the practice. Start with where you are. If the steps for the pose say to lift both arms and you can lift only one, follow your body and lift only one. The variations that follow are suggestions to try that assist an arm or leg in need.

### Bend

If holding your arms out in a T position or raising them overhead triggers tremors or other involuntary movements, try bending that elbow. Also, if a straight-legged position causes spasms, try bending your knees slightly, taking the weight in your thighs, or quadriceps. Try moving gently between these positions, from straight elbow to bent or straightened knees to bent.

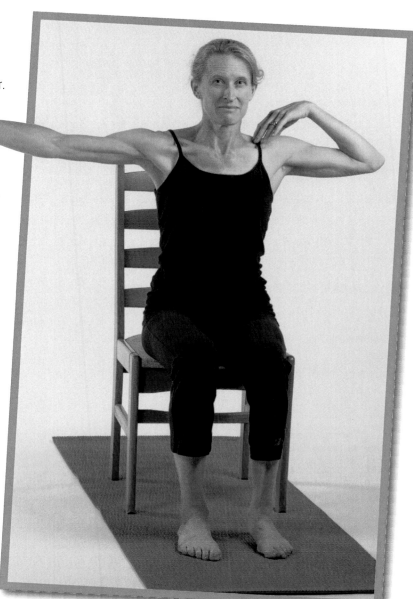

*Bent arm variation*

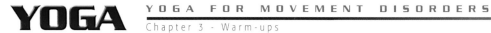

### Strap

Straps, weights and blocks can help if you experience spasms in your legs or feet when seated. Sometimes, simply placing the soles of our feet on the floor trigger pressure points that cramp up toes or arches or cause such tension that your heels bounce involuntarily. Try calming this spasticity by strapping the heel to a block, or weighting the foot with a weight or sandbag or sack of rice.

Also, if your legs tend to flop to one side or the other while you're doing seated upper body poses, you don't have as much support and risk falling. Place a block between your knees and strap your legs together above or below the knees, whichever is more comfortable for you.

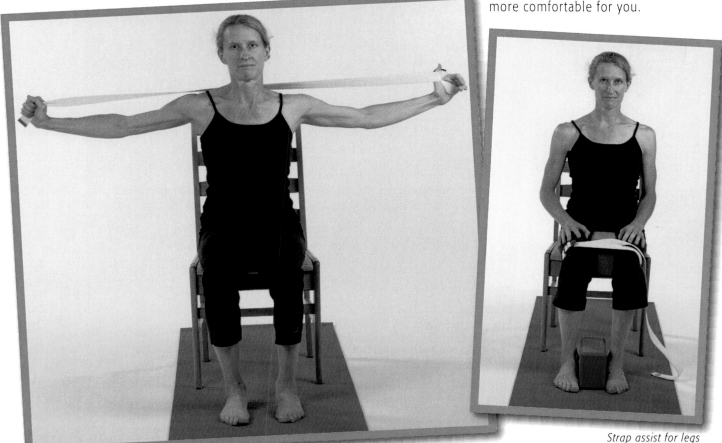

*Strap assist for legs*

*Strap assist for an arm*

### Support

Moving from standing down to the mat can be a daunting task. But lying back brings a deeper relaxation during savasana and in the restorative poses in Chapter 10.  Try using the chair, with some folded blankets for padding if needed, to ease your way down. Start with your chair on the mat to avoid slippage. Face the seat of the chair. Bend forward and place your hands on the edge of the seat and let your arms help you as you kneel onto the mat. Next, sink down to one hip and straighten your legs.

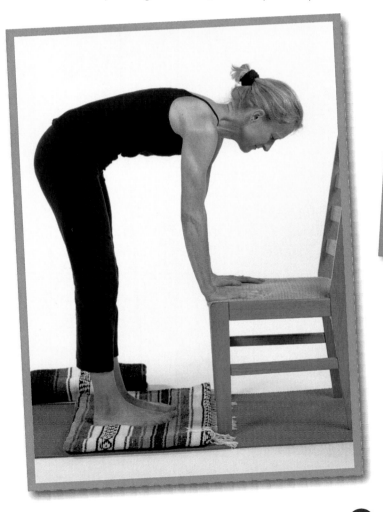

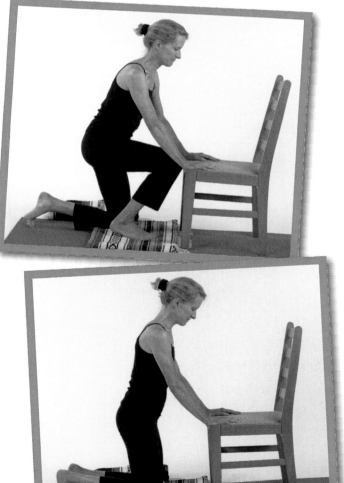

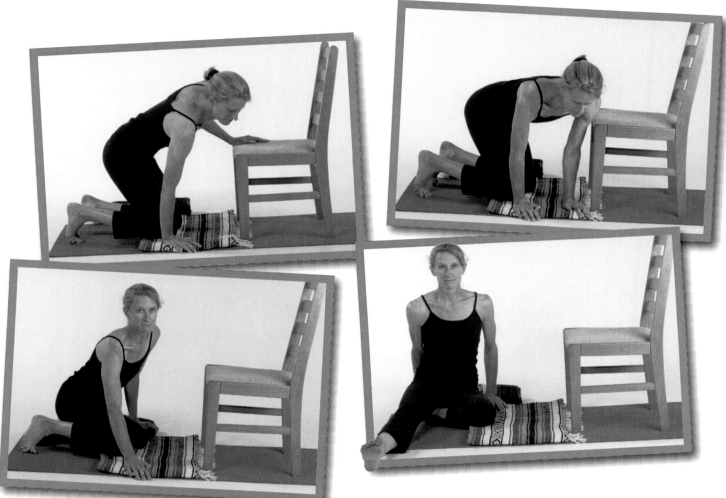

To get back to standing, bend your knees to one side and come up on your knees. Use the chair to help you rise up on your knees. Again, with your arms on the chair for support, bring one foot flat on the mat, followed by the other. Inhale as you straighten your legs.

## Lift
Wheelchair seats can put the spine in a rounded position. To straighten it and bring your hips into a neutral position, try placing a folded or rolled towel beneath your buttocks just behind your sitting bones. Another rolled-up towel placed down the length of your back can help as well.

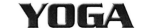

# Part 2

# Practice

## Chapter 4
## SUNDAY: FIND WARMTH

*'Give me the splendid
silent sun...'*
**- Leaves of Grass,
Walt Whitman**

Aging but still spritely, Lasso had trotted around the ring numerous times under the rein of a couple of different young riders at summer camp. By the last lap, the horse was getting ornery. The girl dismounted and tried to lead Lasso to where the next child waited his turn. But he resisted. He'd planted his hooves and refused to move. The girl clucked at him, tugged, pleaded. Tension filled the air as the animal and the girl pulled against one another.

The boy whose turn was next grabbed the reins and tried to yank Lasso to him. The horse held fast. "Wait," the instructor said, slipping the leather straps into her hands and easing close to Lasso. "He needs a minute." She rubbed the gelding's muzzle, scratched behind his ears, and stroked his neck. All the while, she cooed to him, whispering his praises. And when she stepped back, he took a step forward.

That, I thought, watching from the gate, is yoga.

Be gentle. Be kind. Speak with compassion, and your body will respond. Give it warmth and it will glow. What a good way to begin the week.

### ASANA PRACTICE

The sun salutation, or Suryanamaskar, is to many the heart of asana flows. The sun salutations work major joints, inviting synovial fluids that lubricate and cleanse. They also flex and extend the spine, creating warmth. While most yoga poses are about opposing forces, stretching up and down, reaching forward and back, they're also about the balance in this duality. Sun salutations greet the sun and bow to the earth, celebrating our presence in between the two. They can be an energizing way to begin the day or start out the week. They're also a wonderful way to honor the sun's glow, the earth's solidity, our own radiance and strength.

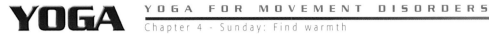
## Coming to Stillness

Find a comfortable yet straight-backed position on a cushion on the mat or in a chair, with your palms resting on your knees or with your hands on a pillow in your lap.

Inhale deeply. Exhale deeply.

Let your eyes drift closed. Imagine you're outside on a cool, overcast day when, for a moment, the clouds dissipate and clear blue sky is unveiled.

Imagine a sunbeam shining on your face. Let it warm you, let it melt away the furrows in your brow and the clench in your jaw. Feel the heat on your skin and let your worries, your clouds, drift away.

Relax in your breathing and warmth for another minute.

## Warm-ups

Please refer to Chapter three for the warm-up exercises to do before practicing the following flow. Work through all of Set A and pose 1 from Set B.

## Poses

## SUN SALUTATION
*Seated Variation*

> *Needed: Straight-backed chair*
> *Sticky mat*
> *Blocks (optional)*

**Difficulty: Any level can enjoy this version.**

1. Sit in mountain pose.

2. **Upward salute:**
   Inhale as you slowly raise both arms to the sky, palms facing upward. If it feels comfortable and you feel stable, have a look up at your hands.

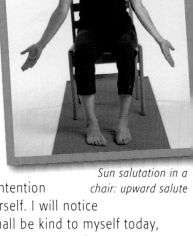

   - Exhale as you reach your arms back slightly, creating an arch in your upper back. This is a nice position to state an intention or affirmation to yourself. I will notice the sun today, or I shall be kind to myself today, or whatever it is that warms you today.

*Sun salutation in a chair: upward salute*

   - Inhale back to straight, arms still reaching to the sky.

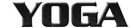
3. **Forward bend:** Exhale as you slowly bend forward, hinging at the hips rather than the waist, and dropping your hands to your thighs. If it feels comfortable, let your torso rest on your thighs, or, drop between your knees. Let your hands rest flat on the mat or on blocks beside your feet.

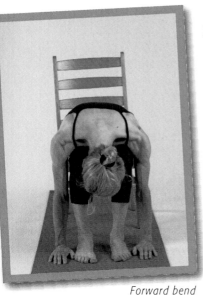

*Forward bend*

4. **Cobra:** Inhale as you push away from your thighs with your hands, pressing your naval forward and your tailbone back. If it feels comfortable, lift your chin slightly.

*Cobra*

5. Exhale and on an inhale, straighten back to seated mountain.

6. **Seated lunge:** Turn to sit sideways on the chair. Bend the front knee at a right angle and lengthen the back leg while reaching up with the crown of your head.

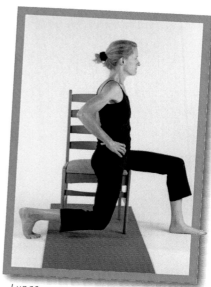

*Lunge*

7. Bring your legs and torso back to seated mountain facing forward.

8. **Seated lunge:** Turn sideways n your chair facing the other and repeat steps 6 and 7.

9. Turn to sit facing forward again. Inhale into an upward salute.

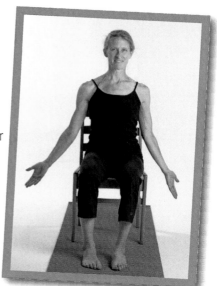

*Upward salute*

10. Exhale your hands down into prayer position over your heart.

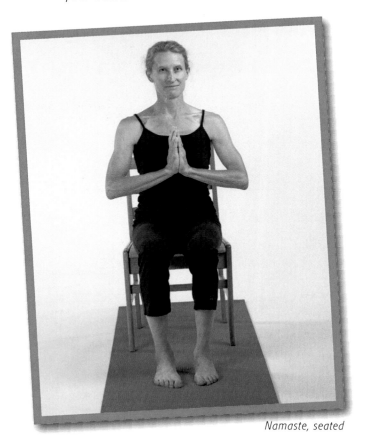

*Namaste, seated*

11. Take a resting breath. Feel your heart with the backs of your thumbs. If you stated an intention or affirmation, this is a nice time to repeat it to yourself.

12. Move into the Relaxation that follows.

## SUN SALUTATION
*Chair-supported Variation*

*Needed: Straight-backed chair*
*Sticky mat*

**Difficulty: The chair provides support, but this is still an energizing flow. If you're new to yoga and exercise or if you get overheated easily, try the seated variation first.**

Place a chair on one end of your mat, the seat facing toward you as you stand in the center of the remaining mat. Be sure the legs of the chair are all on the mat, to prevent it from slipping.

1. Stand in mountain pose facing the chair, a few inches away from it.

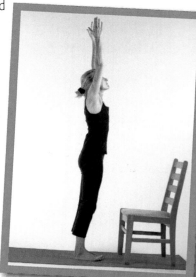

2. **Upward salute:** Inhale as you slowly raise both arms to the sky, palms facing upward. If it feels comfortable and you feel stable, have a look up at your hands.

*Sun salutation chair supported: upward salute*

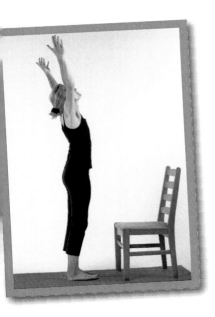

- Exhale as you reach your arms back slightly, creating an arch in your upper back. This is a nice position to state an intention or affirmation to yourself. I will notice the sun today, or I shall be kind to myself today, or whatever it is that warms you today.

- Inhale back to straight, arms still reaching to the sky.

3. **Forward bend:** Exhale as you slowly bend forward, hinging at the hips rather than the waist, and dropping your hands to the chair. As you fold forward, bend your knees as generously as you need to for stability and so there is no strain on your lower

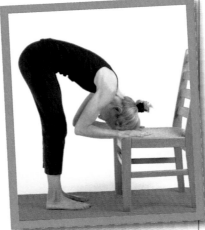

*Forward bend*

back or hamstrings. Bow your head. If it feels comfortable, let the crown of your head touch down lightly on the chair.

4. **Lunge:** Inhale and exhale as you step one leg back straight, bending your front leg.

   a. To prevent injury to your front knee, be sure your thigh and shin and your shin and foot are at right angles.

   b. Lean into your hands to lengthen your back leg as you push the heel down to the mat. Breathe!

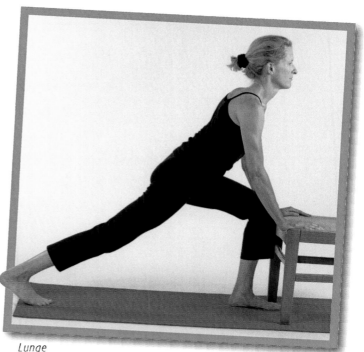

*Lunge*

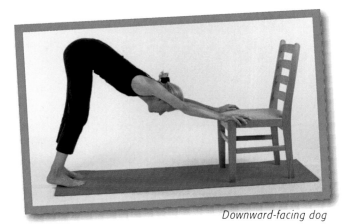

*Downward-facing dog*

5. **Downward-facing dog:** Exhale as you step your other leg back to meet the first one.

   a. Press away from the chair with your hands and reach your tailbone back, hinging at the hips as your head drops so your ears are in line with your arms. Bend your knees slightly, or more if needed.

   b. Keep pressing your tailbone back as you reach the crown of your head toward the seat of the chair.

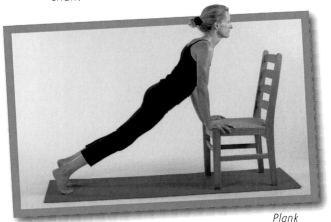

*Plank*

6. **Plank:** Inhale as you pull your hips and abdomen forward, letting your arms and feet bear the weight as your body straightens.

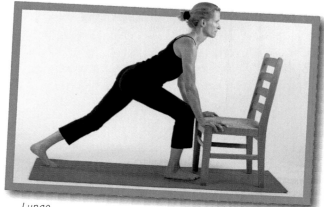

*Lunge*

7. Exhale back to downward-facing dog.

8. Inhale as you step one leg forward into a lunge. Exhale.

9. Inhale as you step the other leg forward into a forward bend. Roll up into mountain pose.

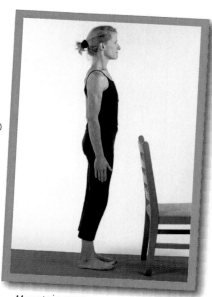

*Mountain pose*

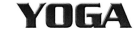

10. Inhale into an upward salute. Exhale your arms to your sides and take a resting breath in mountain pose.

11. Repeat steps 1 through 3.

12. Repeat lunge in step 4 but reach back with the other leg this time, and continue through step 9.

13. Inhale into an upward salute.

14. Exhale your hands down into prayer position over your heart.

15. Take a resting breath. Feel your heart with the backs of your thumbs. If you stated an intention or affirmation, this is a nice time to repeat it to yourself.

16. Move into the Relaxation that follows.

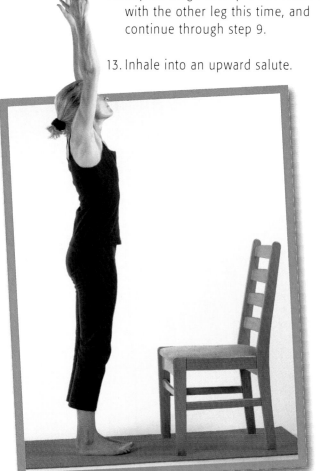

*Upward salute*

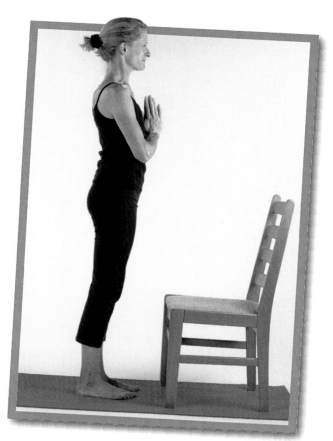

*Namaste*

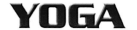

## SUN SALUTATION
*Wall-supported Standing Variation*

*Need: Sticky mat*

Difficulty: Challenging if you have balance concerns. Also, this is an energizing flow. If your MS symptoms include overheating, try the seated variation listed before this. This version does not include a forward bend. Note: If you are avoiding forward bends, this may be a sun salutation that you can try because it does not include a forward bend.

   Spread your mat so the short end is against a wall. Ideally, spread the mat near a corner where there's another wall arm's length away. This could help if you need to reach out for balance. If you're fearful of falling, please use the Seated Variation first.

1.  Stand in mountain pose facing the wall, eight inches to a foot away from it.

2.  **Upward salute:** Inhale as you slowly raise both arms to the sky, palms facing upward. If it feels comfortable and you feel stable, have a look up at your hands.

   •  Exhale as you reach your arms back slightly, creating an arch in your upper back.

   •  Inhale back to straight, arms still open to the sky. This is a nice position to state an intention or affirmation to yourself. I will notice the sun

today, or I shall be kind to myself today, or whatever it is that warms you today.

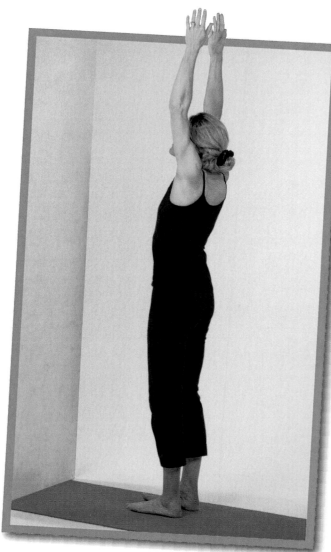

*Sun salutation at wall: upward salute*

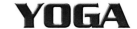
3. **Lunge:** Exhale as you place your hands on the wall at shoulder level and step your right leg back straight, bending your front leg.

   • To prevent injury to your front knee, be sure your thigh and shin and your shin and foot are at right angles.

   • Lean into your hands to lengthen your back leg as you push the heel down to the mat.

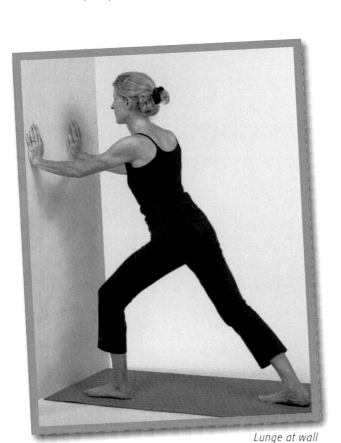

*Lunge at wall*

4. **Half downward-facing dog:** Exhale as you step your left leg back to meet the right.

   • Push away with your hands, reaching your tailbone back and hinging at the hips until your back is parallel to the floor and makes a right angle with your legs. Engage your quads, pulling the knees up (but not locking them). Raise your hands on the wall slightly if your hamstrings are tight or you feel any twinge in your lower back.

   • Keep pressing your tailbone back as you reach the crown of your head toward the wall.

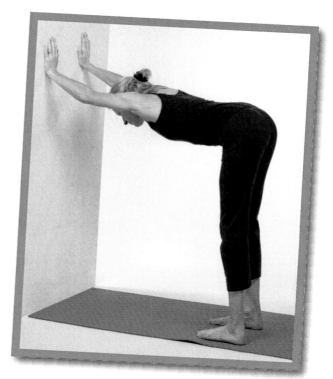

*Half dog*

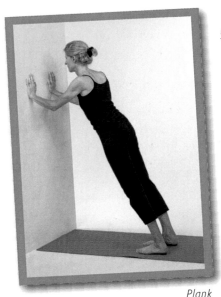

*Plank*

5. **Plank:** Inhale as you pull your hips and abdomen forward, letting your arms and feet bear the weight as your body straightens.

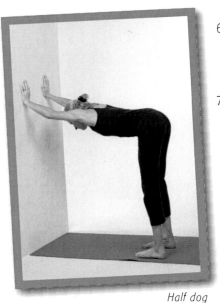

*Half dog*

6. Exhale back to half downward-facing dog.

7. Inhale as you step the right leg forward into a lunge. Exhale.

8. Inhale as you step the left leg forward and roll up into mountain pose.

9. Inhale into an upward salute. Exhale your arms to your sides and take a resting breath in mountain pose.

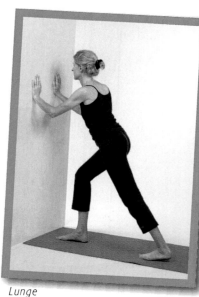

*Lunge*

10. Repeat steps 2 through 9 but reach back with the left leg in lunge.

11. Inhale into an upward salute.

12. Exhale your hands down into prayer position over your heart.

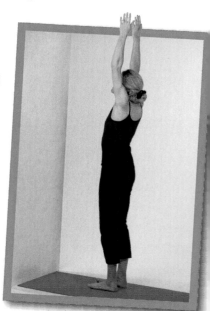

*Upward salute*

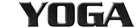
13. Take a resting breath. Feel your heart with the backs of your thumbs. If you stated an intention or affirmation, this is a nice time to repeat it to yourself.

14. Move into the Relaxation that follows.

## RELAXATION: GUIDED IMAGERY

Lie in a comfortable position, warmed by blankets and supported by pillows or bolsters as needed.
An eye pillow (remove glasses or contact lenses first) may be soothing in this guided imagery exercise.

Take a deep breath in. On the exhale, release tension, negative thoughts, planning, to-do lists.

Imagine that you're on a beach, your favorite beach or one you create for yourself in your mind. With ease, you settle onto the sand.

Feel the sun on your face. It is not a burning sun; it is warm. Remember it from before the warm-ups? Let its warmth penetrate your skin. Feel the heat on your sleeves, your arms and shoulders. Let them soften into the sand that has shaped itself to the contours of your body, supporting your head, back, legs. Relax into the sand as the sun warms you.

There's a light breeze on this beach. Allow the air to dance on your skin. Smell the sea in the breeze. Listen to the sounds it brings, the waves gently lapping on shore. In and out. Match your breath to the rhythm of the waves. Allow the in breath to bring with it all that is good. Bring that goodness into your being .Exhale out anything that does not nurture you. Let it go out to sea with the outgoing waves. Inhale and feel all that is good permeate through you just as the sun has.

Warm, supported. Nurtured. The sun is shining, the breeze dancing, the waves moving in and out. Rhythmically. Peacefully. Rhythmically. Peacefully.

Lie on this peaceful beach for several more moments.

Before opening your eyes, begin to bring your awareness back to the room, to your body, to the moment. Wiggle your fingers and toes in the sand, wrinkle your nose up at the sun.

Smile. Know that you can go to this beach, this place of peace at any time. It is yours.

May the warm sun shine upon you. May love surround you. May peace fill you. Namaste.

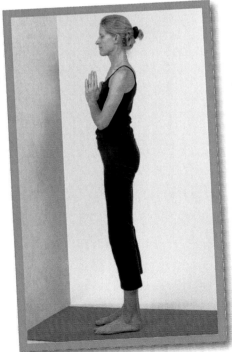

*Namaste*

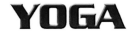
## ESPECIALLY BENEFICIAL

- With some movement disorders, our voices can soften. The upward salute increases the space between our ribs where the intercostal muscles are that help us breathe, allowing for more oxygen when we inhale. Good lung capacity can result in stronger voice projection.

- Upward salute and forward bend can loosen the cervical disks and surrounding ligaments of the neck, which can become particularly stiff.

- Weight-bearing on the shoulder muscles in half dog or down dog helps to strengthen the upper body, this can be useful when turning in bed at night.

- Falling can be a concern with the muscle weakness and imbalance that accompany Parkinson's, MS, stroke, and other disorders. Weight-bearing on the shoulders aids in building strong bones so we don't break anything if we do stumble.

- The iliopsoas muscle (made up of two connecting muscles) runs from the upper thigh at the head of the femur around to the lower spine. This major muscle can get overly rigid, not only affecting our gait in walking but also tweaking the lower back. Lunges help stretch and release this muscle.

## YOGA TO GO: APPLYING IT TO YOUR DAY

- Go outside. Sit or hold onto a railing for balance. Close your eyes and turn your face up toward the sun for a minute or two. Take a deep breath and feel the warmth.

- Watch a sunrise. Notice the changes in color, in the air.

- Watch a sunset. Watch another one a day or two later and note how it's different.

- Take a nap near a sunny window. Rest and restore in the glow.

- Say something kind to yourself.

- Release your spine before bed. Forward bends can be calming to the nervous system. Before turning in at night, sit on the edge of the bed and gently bend forward, hinging at the hips with a straight back (place your hands on your thighs for support). Then let your back curl before slowly rolling back up. This may help with sleep.

- Stretch your spine in the morning. Back extensions (or, arching back) are said to stimulate the nervous system. A soft, easy back extension like in an upward salute might shake off drowsiness in the morning.

- Move into half downward-facing dog (Step 4 of the Wall-supported Standing Variation) at the kitchen sink, the bathroom counter, in the aisle on an airplane for a spine awakener.

- Take yourself to the beach, literally or figuratively, using the beach in your mind's eye from the relaxation. Either way, get to the beach. Often.

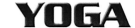
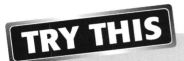

### EYE PILLOWS ON HAND

It can be a challenge to soften muscles during Relaxation when fists are involuntarily clenched, or the tremor in one arm won't let it rest. Try this: Place an eye pillow or light sand bag in your palms to help alleviate the tension (even if it's only one hand that needs the weight, it's a nice balance to place one in each palm). In cool temperatures, store the eye pillows on a radiator or heat vent so that they are warm for relaxation time.

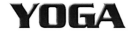
# Chapter 5
# MONDAY: FEEL THE PULL

'Well, it's a marvelous night
for a moondance'.
– Moondance ,Van Morrison

When Danielle was a little girl, she used to believe that the man in the moon lived and danced in a marshmallow house.

It started when her mother commented on the moon one night while driving home. Danielle peered out the back of the station wagon to see for herself. Her mother learned years later that Danielle thought she'd been pointing at the city water tower, which, to a four year old, looked like an ideal place for the moon to live: in a marshmallow on sticks.  It was no wonder the man in the moon was dancing.

Danielle remembers that even when she was too far away to see the marshmallow tower, she never doubted the moon's presence. She was right. A full moon lures anyone looking up at it into romance and poetry. But even when the night sky is dark, the moon's force still sways moods and tugs at the tides.

A similar energy exists with yoga, even when we're not looking. Yoga has a poetic power of its own: the mind/body connection. Gaze into it and see. Let it pull you in to dance.

## ASANA PRACTICE

The moon series, or chandra namaskar, is cooling and a good way to end the day. Or, move through the series at any time of day, particularly if you're trying not to overheat, as is often the case with MS, or, at times when tone or tremor is particularly active.

Like the sun salutation, moon poses invite opposing forces to work while maintaining a balanced center. This asana flow focuses on strengthening and stretching the muscles that allow the legs to kick forward and back and turn in and out – the hip flexors and extenders as well as the adductors and abductors.

The poses in this series resemble the moon as it moves through its phases. But know, too, that they also work the legs. To avoid fatigue, try only the first three steps for a few weeks. When you feel comfortable proceeding through the series, pause at any time, particularly between steps, to take a resting breath.

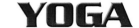

There are numerous variations on the moon series.

In each, the flow reaches to the sky while solidly grounded. As the moon spreads an even glow, reflecting the light of the sun, this flow can create a calming way to shine from within.

### Coming to stillness
Find a comfortable, straight-backed position on a cushion, on the mat or in a chair, with your palms resting on your knees or with your hands on a pillow in your lap.

Inhale deeply.

On the next exhale, breathe out anything that is not calming – your to-do list, a mental replay of an argument, pain, the driver who cut you off – exhale it all. Picture your outgoing breath as hot, smoggy, and heavy, like the hazy sun on a sweltering day.

As you inhale, image a pristine lake reflecting the moonrise. Breathe in the cool, crisp, clean night air.

Follow this for two more breaths, relaxing in the image of the white glow on deep, clear water.

### Warm-ups
Please refer to Chapter three for the warm-up exercises to do before practicing the following flow. Work through all of Set A and poses four and five from Set B.

*Poses*

## MOON SERIES
*Seated Variation*

*Need: Sticky mat, Straight-backed chair*
*Blocks, books, or firm blanket (optional)*

**Difficulty: Any level can try this flow.**

Spread your mat and place the chair on a short end, seat facing the mat. Be sure all four legs of the chair are on the mat to prevent slipping. Ideally, spread the mat where there's a wall arm's length away. This could help if you need to reach out for balance.

1. Sit in Seated Mountain pose.

2. **Crescent Moon:** Inhale as you slowly raise both arms to the sky. Clasp fingers, with index fingers pointing up in temple position. Exhale gently to the right, pressing your left hip down into the chair. Keep both feet grounded on

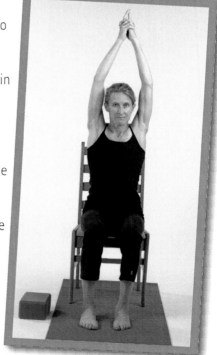

*Moon series in a chair: crescent moon*

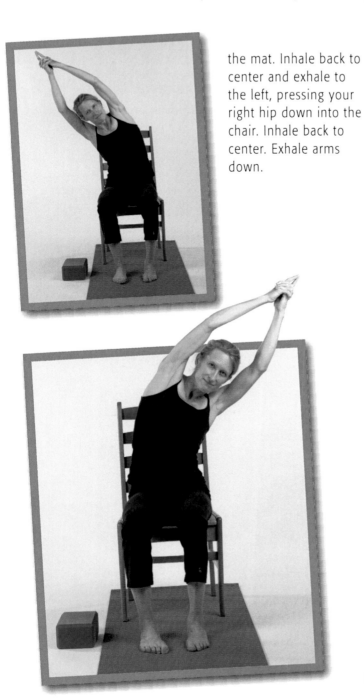

the mat. Inhale back to center and exhale to the left, pressing your right hip down into the chair. Inhale back to center. Exhale arms down.

3. **Goddess:** Step your feet about shoulder-width apart. Inhale and raise your arms to T position then on an exhale, bend your elbows, fingers pointing up and palms facing each other. If this feels comfortable, remain in the pose for an extra breath or two. Release your arms. Shake out your arms and take a resting breath.

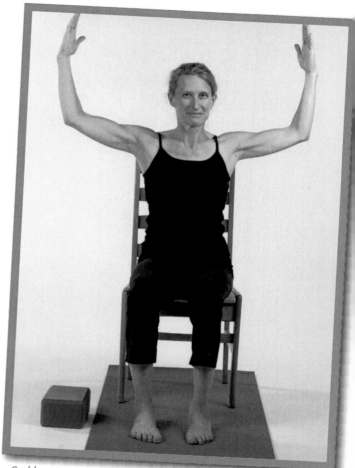

*Goddess*

4. **Seated Forward Bend with Twist:** With a straight back, exhale and hinge forward placing your hands on the floor or on a block. Center your right hand on the block. On an inhale, sweep your left arm up to the sky. If it is comfortable, look up at your fingertips. Exhale and release your arm down and repeat with your right arm.

   • **Optional:** If it is not comfortable for you to reach your arm up, place your right hand on your knee and look over your right shoulder. Repeat for the left side.

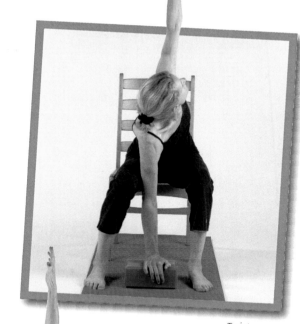

*Twist*

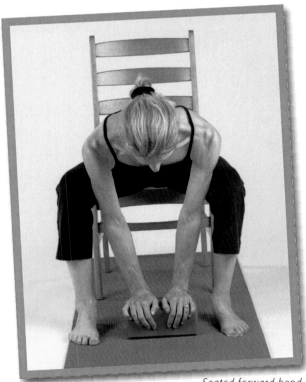

*Seated forward bend*

59

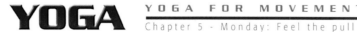

5. **Seated Hamstring Stretch:**
   Come back into seated mountain pose at the edge of your chair. Stretch your right leg straight in front of you, foot flexed, your left leg bent with knee and ankle at 90 degree angles. Place your hands on the chair for support as you exhale and hinge forward from the hips. Feel that your spine is straight, not rounded. If your hamstrings feel especially tight, sit up some. Release back to mountain and switch legs.

   • **Optional:** If your feet don't reach the floor to form a comfortable right angle at the ankle, place your feet on blocks, a phone book or books, or a firm, folded blanket.

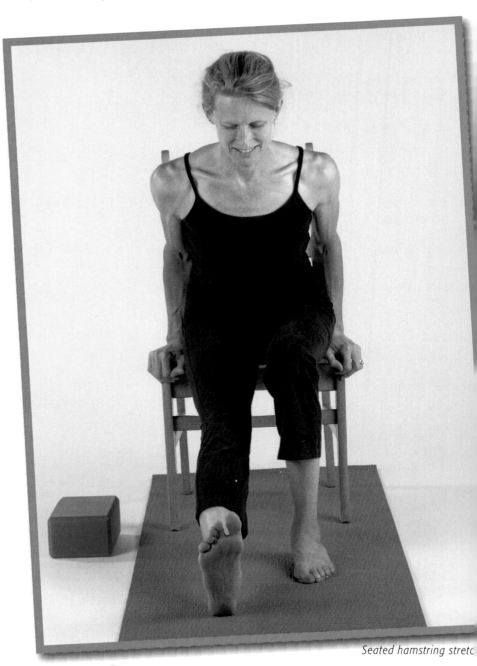

*Seated hamstring stretc*

6. **Goddess:** Reposition yourself in the chair so you are facing forward. Repeat Step 3.

7. **Crescent Moon:** Repeat Step 2.

8. Take a resting breath. Prepare for the Relaxation that follows.

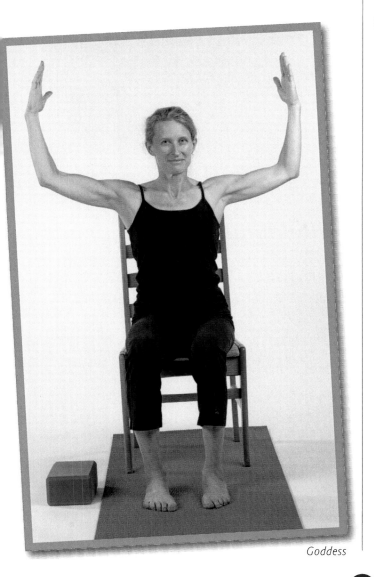

*Goddess*

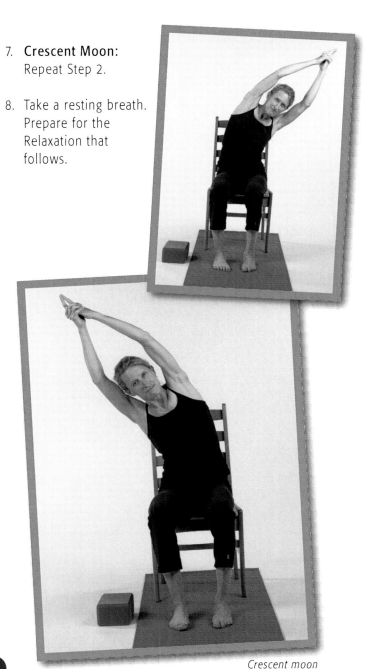

*Crescent moon*

## MOON SERIES
*Supported Standing Variation*

*Need: Sticky mat*
*Straight-backed chair*
*Block*

**Difficulty: This can be a challenging flow if you have balance concerns or are new to stretching. Try the seated variation first.**

Spread your mat and place the chair on a short end of it, the seat facing the mat. Be sure all four legs of the chair are on the mat to prevent slipping. Ideally, spread the mat where there's a wall arm's length away. This could help if you need to reach out for balance. If you're fearful of falling, please use the Seated Variation.

1. Stand in Mountain pose to the left of the seat of the chair, about six inches away from it.

2. **Crescent Moon:** Inhale as you slowly raise both arms to the sky. Clasp fingers, with index fingers pointing up in temple position. Notice if your elbows are straight but not locked. Exhale your upper body gently to the right, allowing your left hip to glide slightly left, but keeping weight even on both feet. Inhale back to center and exhale to the left, allowing your right hip to glide slightly right, weight even on both feet. Inhale back to center. Exhale arms down.

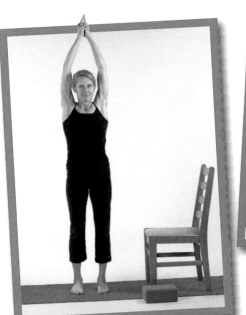

*Moon series standing:*
*crescent moon*

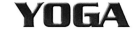

3. **Goddess:** Step your feet about shoulder-width apart, toes pointing outward, about 30 degrees. Bend your knees slightly. (Caution: Be certain that the bent knee is not extending past the ankle; there should be a right angle at the ankle, the knee directly over it. You should be able to see your big toes.) Raise arms to T position then bend elbows, fingers pointing up and palms facing each other. If this feels comfortable, remain in the pose for an extra breath or two.

   a. Try to keep your torso straight, as though a line runs from your nose to your navel to the center point on the mat between your feet.

   b. Feel the contact with the ground through your feet as you reach through your fingertips and crown of your head, keeping your shoulders relaxed.

4. With an inhale, straighten your legs and release your arms to your waist.

5. **Wide angle forward bend:** With a straight back, hinge forward placing your hands on the floor or on a block. Bend your knees if you feel any strain in your lower back or hamstrings.

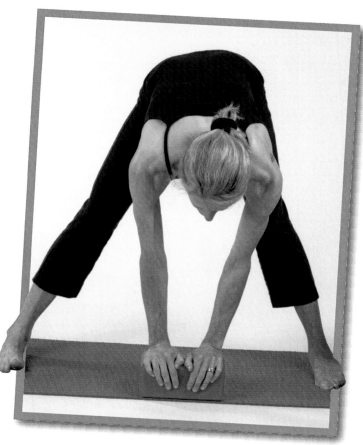

*Wide angle forward bend*

*Goddess*

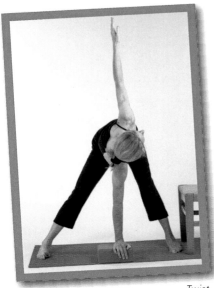

*Twist*

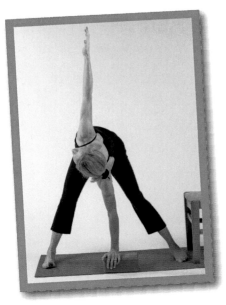

6. **Twist:** Center your right hand on the block. On an inhale, sweep your left arm up to the sky. If it is comfortable, look up at your fingertips. On an exhale, release your arm down and repeat with your right arm.

7. Come back to center, inhaling as you press into your feet and roll back up to standing.

8. **Standing Head to Knee:** Stand and pivot your feet to face the chair. Your right foot is now behind you, your left foot forward. Keeping your legs straight, hinge forward at the hips. Place your hands on the chair and, if possible, bow your head toward your left knee. If your hamstrings feel especially tight, bow your head to the chair seat rather than your knee.

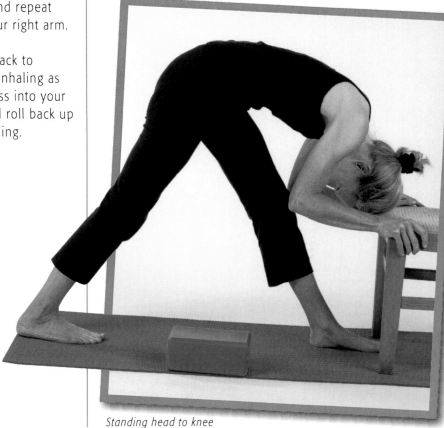

*Standing head to knee*

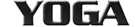

9. **Kneeling Warrior:** From standing head to knee, use the chair support your upper body with your hands as you drop to your right knee, which is slightly behind your hip. Bend the left at 90 degrees. (Caution: Be certain that the bent knee is not extending past the ankle; there should be a right angle at the ankle, the knee stacked directly over it.) You should be able to see the big toe of your left foot.) Use one or both hands on the chair for balance. If you feel balanced, supported by your grounded left foot, leave your left hand on the chair with a light touch and raise your right fingertips to the sky. Breathe into the stretch, allowing your hips to come slightly forward.

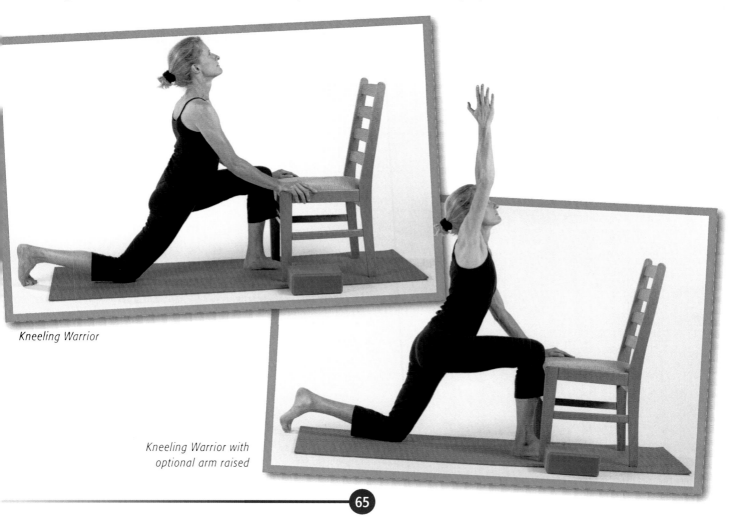

*Kneeling Warrior*

*Kneeling Warrior with optional arm raised*

10. **Switch:** Bring your left knee to the mat then back and your right leg forward, the right foot on the mat and the knee at 90 degrees. If you feel balanced, supported by your grounded right foot and right hand, raise your left fingertips to the sky. Breathe into the stretch in your left thigh's quad and psoas muscles.

11. **Standing Head to Knee:** With your hands on the chair for support, straighten both legs and bow forward as in Step 7.

12. **Wide angle forward bend:** Stand and pivot your feet to the left so you are sideways on the mat. Repeat Step 5, facing the opposite way.

*Standing head to knee*

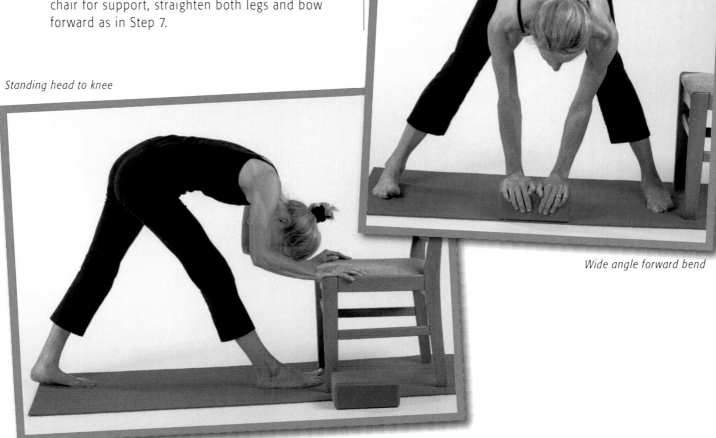

*Wide angle forward bend*

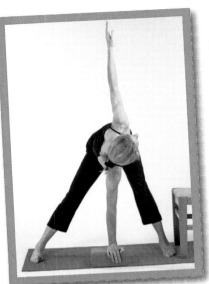

13. **Twist:** Repeat Step 6. Inhale to standing.

*Twist*

15. **Crescent Moon:** Repeat Step 2.

16. Take a resting breath. Prepare for the Relaxation that follows.

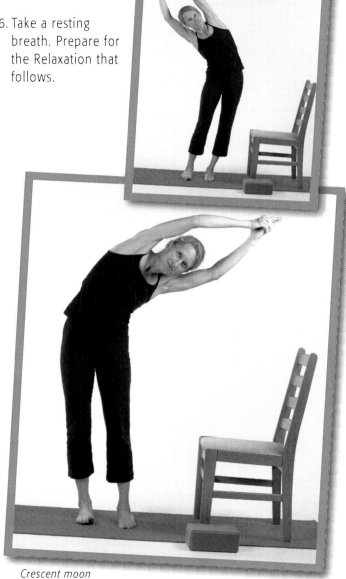

14. **Goddess:** Repeat Step 3.

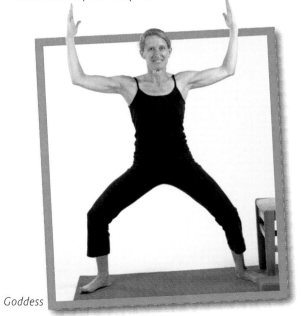

*Goddess*

*Crescent moon*

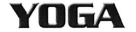

## RELAXATION: GUIDED IMAGERY

Lie or sit, perhaps with legs up on a facing chair, in a comfortable position, warmed by blankets and supported by pillows or bolsters as needed. Again, an eye pillow (remove glasses or contact lenses first) may be soothing in this guided imagery exercise.

Inhale, and then exhale fully. Take a deep breath in to the count of four. Pause to the count of four. Exhale completely. Repeat this one more time before returning to your natural breath. Feel your back supported by the floor or chair back, the back of your shoulders, your upper back, your sacrum and hips.

Recall the moonlight you brought to mind during Coming to Stillness. It's a pure, clean light reflecting off the lake. Let that light enter through the crown of your head, illuminating cells with its cool, healing presence. Watch the light as it moves down into the neck and shoulders, shining into dark corners. Follow the clean, white path it makes as it lights the spine, organs, hips and legs down through the feet and into each toe.

Allow the moonlight reflection to return to the water, breathing in the cool, clear air off the lake. Rest for a few more minutes, supported, cleansed, healing.

Before opening your eyes, begin to bring your awareness back to the room, to your body, to the moment. Wiggle your fingers and toes, wrinkle your nose. And smile. Know that the pure healing light of the moon is always there, even if you can't see it.

May you be supported, as the night sky holds the moon, allowing you to shine through every phase that is you. Namaste.

## ESPECIALLY BENEFICIAL

• Strong, flexible hip/groin muscles support us, help us walk. And dance.

• Stroke recovery can still leave us walking with a limp. Strengthening the legs helps both legs carry the load.

• The uneven gait that comes with a stroke or with movement disorders such as Parkinson's can affect the lower back. Keeping our hamstrings from getting too tight helps take some stress off the lumbar and sacral joints of the back and hips.

• Weight-bearing on the legs in goddess pose can help maintain strong pelvic bones, which can help against developing osteoporosis.

• In Head to Knee, the heart is higher than the brain, creating an inversion of blood flow, which can help create a sense of calm, even sleepiness. Will it cure the insomnia related to movement disorders or side effects of medication? No, but it can help.

## YOGA TO GO: APPLYING IT TO YOUR DAY

• Look at the moon tonight. How much of it can you see? Is it waxing or waning?

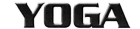

- Check a lunar calendar to see what phases the moon will go through over the next two weeks. Notice what changes you go through in the same timeframe.

- Notice the night air. Breathe it in. Is it heavier or lighter than it was during the day?

- Make note of something that, like yoga or the moon,

is always there for you. Your breath. Your heartbeat. The chance to say something kind to yourself.

- Dance. In the shower, in the kitchen, with someone you love. A study by a team of researchers at Washington University School of Medicine in St. Louis found that the tango helps people with Parkinson's with balance and mobility[3].

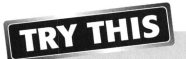

**WAKE-UP YOGA**

A refreshing way to begin the day is with some yoga before getting out of bed. Try this: Lie on your back and take a deep breath in and out. Focus on the air moving from the tip of your nose down into your expanding ribs. Feel your belly rise and then fall with your outgoing breath. Take another inhale and on an exhale, pull one knee to your chest. On the next exhale, pull the other knee up, too. Wrap your arms around your shins, or knees, or wherever they reach, and hug your legs close, without lifting your head. Release, stretch long and take one more full, deep breath. On the exhale: smile. Sometimes this is the only yoga that will fit into the day. Or, maybe you'll greet each day this way. I do.

# Chapter 6
# TUESDAY: TWIST IT

*'And the stars look very different today'.*
*– Space Oddity, David Bowie*

Years ago, before layoffs became commonplace, a group of coworkers received word that the reorganization of the department did not include jobs for them. Cradling their belongings in cardboard boxes, they were gone before colleagues had a chance to say good-bye. We wondered what the future held for them, especially Ron. He'd worked there for decades and had earned a senior position. Why Cathy? She was the go-to assistant who knew where everything was filed and stored.

Over the course of time, a shift happened in Ron and Cathy. Ron immersed himself in hospice work, talking little about what he used to do and more about the connections he was feeling. Cathy let her creative side open up and won numerous awards in graphic arts.

Ron and Cathy didn't lose their identities when they lost their jobs. Stripped of the exterior labels, they discovered who they were within. Practicing yoga can do just this. It turns us inward to self-reflect, not to look at what we do but at who we are.

## ASANA PRACTICE

Twist poses wring out the muscles along the spine, releasing tension caught there. In turn, the motion can soothe tension caught elsewhere: in our minds. When we practice twisting poses, we rotate like a barbershop sign, spiraling from, and back, to the starting point: ourselves.

In a twist, we can reflect and take a moment to recoil before springing back into the action of daily living. But, remember to be gentle. Twists are not about how far we go into the stretch. Move to where your body allows, to where you feel it is today, not to where you think it should be.

### Coming to stillness
Sit in a comfortable, straight-backed position in a chair, with your palms resting on your knees or with your hands on a pillow in your lap.

Inhale deeply. Feel the air enter, from the tip of the nose down the back of your throat. Notice if breath comes in at the top or bottom of the nasal passage. Is the air warm or cool?

Exhale deeply. Notice if the breath exits at the top or bottom of the nasal passage. Is it warm or cool?

Rub your palms together briskly to warm your palms. Once warmed, place your cupped palms gently over

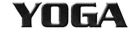

your closed eyes. Feel the heat through your eyelids. Let your hands block out light, tension, to-do lists. Breathe deeply for another minute this way.

## Warm-ups

Please refer to Chapter three for the warm-up exercises to do before practicing the following flow. Work through all of Set A and poses two and seven (if you're comfortable standing) from Set B.

## Poses

If you have any concern about falling from the chair in these poses, particularly when there is a forward bend, place your chair facing a wall. Reach out to the wall for balance at any time.

Gentle twists can alleviate back pain. Sometimes, any kind of twist can sometimes aggravate back pain. Should you experience discomfort or pain in your back during a twist, come out of the pose.

## TWIST
*Seated Twist*

*Need: Straight-backed chair, Sticky mat*

**Difficulty: Any level can try this pose.**

This asana gently spirals up from the base to the top of the spine.

1. Sit sideways on the chair, feet on the floor with ankles at a 90-degree angle (add a blanket or cushion beneath your feet if your legs aren't long enough for your feet to rest this way).

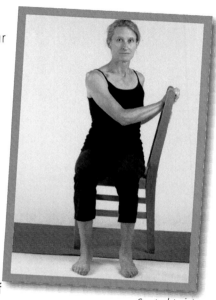

*Seated twist*

2. Place both hands on the back of the chair, very lightly gripping it.

3. Inhaling, lengthen your spine by pressing up through the crown of your head and down with your sitting bones into the chair.

4. Exhaling, twist at your base, turning your abdomen toward the back of the chair.

5. Inhaling, lengthen your spine.

6. Exhaling, twist at your middle, turning your rib cage toward the back of the chair.

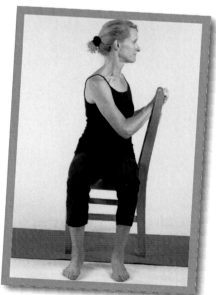

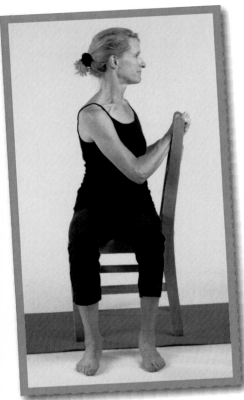

You can gently use your arms assist in the twist.

7. Inhaling, lengthen your spine.

8. Exhaling, twist at your shoulders.

9. Inhaling, lengthen your spine.

10. Exhaling, turn your neck toward the back of the chair and gaze over your shoulder.

11. To come out of the twist, release your hands and gently uncoil.

12. Take a resting breath before sitting sideways in the other direction on the chair, following the steps to twist on that side.

13. Take a resting breath before moving to the next asana.

## TWIST
*Standing Twist at Wall*

*Need: Straight-backed chair, armless chair*

**Difficulty: Anyone who can stand comfortably can try this pose.**

This pose can help with fatigue.

1. Position your chair with the back against a wall. Stand with your right shoulder touching the wall and step your right leg onto the chair.

2. Place your palms on the wall.

3. Inhale and press down through both feet, extending up through the crown of your head.

4. Exhale and turn toward the wall, using your hands for support.

5. Stay in the twist for several seconds, working up to a minute over time.

6. Stepping your right foot back down, take a moment to shake out both arms and legs.

7. Stand on the other side of the chair with your left shoulder touching the wall and repeat on the left side.

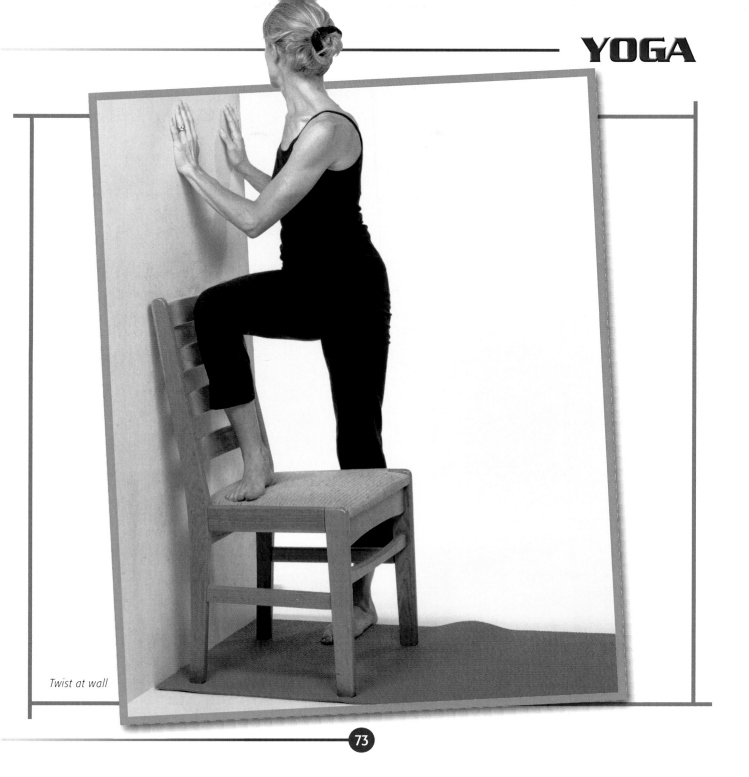

Twist at wall

## TWIST
*Cross-legged Twist*

*Need: Mat*
*Blanket or cushion or bolster*
*Blocks (optional)*

**Difficulty: Anyone who doesn't have difficulty getting to the floor comfortably can try this pose.**

This pose helps release the lower back.

1. Sit cross-legged on the mat. Use a folded blanket or cushion or bolster to raise your sitting bones so your back is straight and your hips are positioned slightly forward. The higher you are seated, the easier it is to sit with a straight back. If your back is rounded, even on the bolster, skip this asana and prepare for the Relaxation that follows.

2. Place cushions or blocks under your knees for support, particularly if your groin muscles are tight.

3. Place your right hand on your left knee.

4. Inhale as you lengthen up and exhale as you twist from the abdomen to the left.

5. Lighten the pressure into your right sitting bone as you twist, keeping the hip free to follow the movement.

6. Inhale as you lengthen up and exhale as you continue the twist from the ribs and, with the next two rounds of breath, from the shoulders and head.

7. Untwist and repeat on the left side.

8. Untwist and take a resting breath.

9. Prepare for Relaxation that follows. Use a folded blanket for a pillow, another blanket over you for warmth.

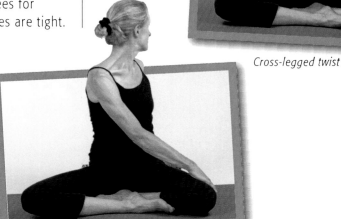

*Cross-legged twist*

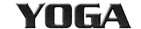

## RELAXATION: GUIDED IMAGERY

Lie in a comfortable position, warmed by blankets and supported by pillows or bolsters as needed. Again, an eye pillow (remove glasses or contact lenses first) may be soothing in this guided imagery exercise.

Inhale deeply and release the breath with an audible sigh. Prepare to go to a favorite place – a cabin in the woods, your childhood home – a place that's warm and comfortable and safe.

Drive there in a sporty car or ride on horseback or on the wings of a bird. When you get there, find a spot to lie down and relax. Settle in.

What colors are there in your favorite place?

What do you hear there?
Birdsong? Laughter?

Can you smell the ocean?
Or new-mown grass?

What is your favorite treat there?
Can you taste it?

What do your fingers reach out and touch?
Sand? The velvet fur of a dog's ear?

For several minutes, relax into this safe, warm, comfortable place with all your senses.

Before opening your eyes, begin to bring your awareness back to the room, to your body, to the moment. Wiggle your fingers and toes, wrinkle your nose. Take a deep breath in – maybe you can still smell the scents of your favorite place. Exhale knowing you can go back to this place anytime, not to do anything there but to safely be who you are.

May you be at peace. Namaste.

## ESPECIALLY BENEFICIAL

- Our trunk muscles around the waist and hips get tight with various movement disorders. Twists help release the grip.

- With an uneven gait, particularly if a stroke has affected the nerves on one side of the body, the lower back can get strained. Twists help reset the vertebrae and muscle fibers to relieve that strain.

- If you drive, being able to turn to look behind you is safer than relying solely on the rearview mirror.

- Parkinson's can cause a stoop when standing and the imbalance in muscle strength from a stroke or MS affects how straight we stand. Twists can help our posture by releasing tightness in the back and by strengthening the shoulders and arms as they assist in the movement.

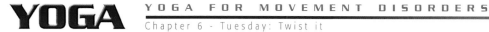

YOGA TO GO: APPLYING IT TO YOUR DAY

- Webster's Dictionary defines layoff as a period of inactivity or idleness. Each day, layoff something on your to-do list. Breathe and be for those few moments.

- Typically, when someone asks us what we do, we respond by switching to the verb form of be. I am a vet, gardener, student. The next time, answer using the verb do. Notice if that changes how you identify who you are.

- If you sit for long periods – at a desk, in the car – and your back feels tight, twist it. Airplanes are an especially good place to twist. Restaurants can be, too.

TRY THIS

TAP DANCE

When all the concentration you can muster still doesn't get some body part to move, try this: tap. Specifically, lightly touch the part you want to move with the tips of your fingers. For example, if you're turning in bed from your side to your stomach, tap on back of the hip. It doesn't work every time, but often it does. Tapping helps the brain make the connection to the muscles that internal chemistry isn't doing.

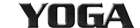
# Chapter 7
# WEDNESDAY: FOLLOW YOUR BREATH

'Let it be'.
– The Beatles

Despite the stickers on the glass, birds still fly across my back deck into the sliding doors. A female grosbeak hit hard one summer day. She landed belly up, her chest rising and falling in quick breaths.

I ached to scoop her up in a towel and take her to the nearby sanctuary for injured wild birds. I knew not to interfere, though. Not yet. Give it a little time. Besides her breathing, all that moved were her eyes, and I sensed she saw me looking at her. It was an unnatural sight, her underside exposed, legs sprawled. I felt like I'd caught a glimpse of someone behind a hospital curtain, pale and mouth agape.

Busying myself in the kitchen, I put dishes away as though my doing an everyday task would help the bird get back to normal. I checked her again. She'd righted herself, but was crooked and quite still but for her breathing. I found another chore to do before glancing out at her again. Still crooked, still breathing. I opened mail, made a sandwich. Still on the deck but still breathing. Thinking it might be time to wrap her in the towel, I looked out again. She was gone.

The stunned bird hadn't sung out. She didn't stretch a wing. Instinctually, she simply breathed. Wherever our yoga journeys take us – to sun salutations atop a mountain peak or restorative poses in the comfort of our own rooms – we must breathe. It centers us, brings healing. Breathe and we can soar.

## ASANA PRACTICE

Beyond asana practice, there is also breathing practice or pranayama. Prana means breath and includes the life energy that fills us as we breathe. Pranayama translates as regulating the breath, or, loosely, breathing exercises.

Notice your breathing when someone cuts you off in traffic. It becomes short, shallow, carrying little oxygen and signaling stress to the rest of the body. Notice your breathing when you're enjoying a good book. It is more rhythmic, deeper, letting the body know there's no need for alarm. By focusing on our breath, we can bring an awareness to what's going on in our bodies as well as our minds.

### Coming to stillness
Find a comfortable, straight-backed position on a cushion, on the mat or in a chair, with your palms resting on your knees. Take three regular breaths.

On the next inhalation, place your hands on your belly. Breathe in and let your belly press into your palms. Feel your hands sink in as you exhale.

Place your hands on your rib cage. Breathe into your belly and, taking in a bit more air let it expand your ribs. Exhale, pushing the air out with your belly first, then letting your ribs drop down as you continue your exhale.

Bring your fingertips to your upper chest, just beneath your collar bones. Breathe in and expand your belly, your ribs, and then your upper chest. Feel your fingertips rise with the inhale. Exhale. Pushing the air out, feel your upper chest lower, your rib cage drop, your belly contract.

Breathe this way for one more cycle of breath, and imagine inhaling good, nurturing energy and exhaling out anything that is stale or negative.

### Warm-ups

Please refer to Chapter three for the warm-up exercises to do before practicing the following breathing exercises. Work through all of Set A.

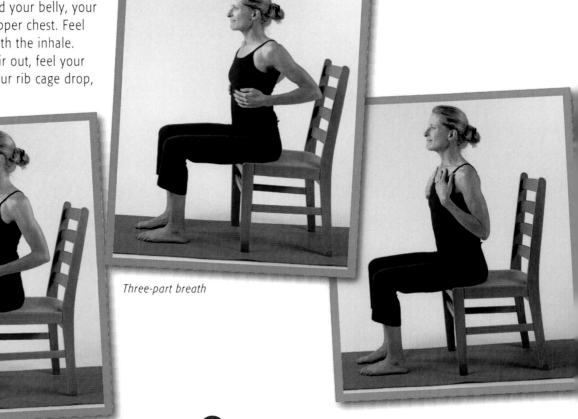

*Three-part breath*

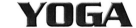
*Poses*

Breath control can be energizing or calming, depending on the pattern of breathing. By changing our breathing pattern, we can alter that state and the stresses it has on our bodies.

**BREATH EXERCISES**

*Bee breath or Humming breath*

*Need: Straight-backed chair*

**Difficulty: Anyone can try this exercise.**

This breathing exercise can be helpful for anxiety. For added centering, try using earplugs and/or closing your eyes.

1. Sit comfortably on your sitting bones. Lengthen your spine by pressing your sitting bones down into the chair as you reach up through the crown of your head.

2. Inhale fully through your nose.

3. With mouth closed, jaw relaxed, make a humming sound as you exhale. Notice if the vibration is in the roof of your mouth and cheekbones.

4. Breathe this way for three more cycles of breath.

5. Inhale again through your nose.

6. Press your back teeth together gently and make a humming sound as you exhale. Notice if the vibration moves to your sinuses and vertebrae in your neck.

**BREATH EXERCISES**

*Lion's breath*

*Need: Straight-backed chair*

**Difficulty: Anyone can try this exercise.**

This is a calming breathing exercise.

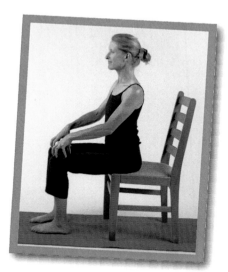

1. Sit comfortably on your sitting bones. Lengthen your spine by pressing your sitting bones down into the chair as you reach up through the crown of your head.

2. Place your hands on your knees, fingers curled like claws.

3. Let your mouth open.

4. As you inhale, tilt your head back slightly, opening your mouth wider.

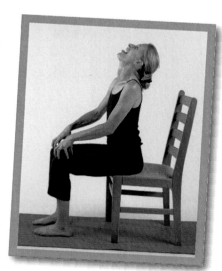

*Lion's breath*

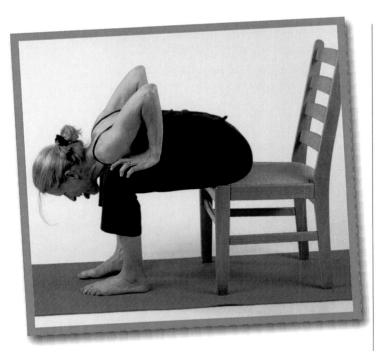

5. Hinge forward at the hips, sticking your tongue out and exhaling from your throat with an audible haaa.

6. Close your mouth and on an inhale, straighten back up to a seated position.

7. Relax your hands palms-down on your lap and take a resting breath.

8. Repeat steps 2 through 7 two more times, imaging that you are spilling any anger, frustration, negative thoughts into the earth through your open mouth as you exhale.

**BREATH EXERCISES**
*Counting breath*

*Need: Straight-backed chair*

**Difficulty: Anyone can try this exercise.**

This exercise helps focus the mind and settle thoughts. It can be useful before meditation or sleep.

1. Sit comfortably on your sitting bones. Lengthen your spine by pressing your sitting bones down into the chair as you reach up through the crown of your head.

2. Inhale halfway to the count of four.

3. Pause your breath to the count of four.

4. Inhale the rest of your breath to the count of four.

5. Pause to the count of four.

6. Slowly exhale completely.

7. Repeat several more times, noticing your belly expand and contract with the inhales and exhales.

8. Prepare for Relaxation that follows.

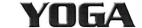

## RELAXATION: GUIDED IMAGERY

Lie with props as needed under your head and neck, knees, with your back comfortable. Let the blankets and props fully support you.

Breathe regularly and listen to the sounds around you. A car driving down the street, perhaps, or a fan running. Next, listen to the sound of your breath. How quiet can you make it?

Follow that sound inside as your breath expands your belly and ribs. Do you hear anything in your body? An ache, a twinge? Send your breath to any spaces needing expanding or calming.

Recall the good, nurturing energy you started with during Coming to Stillness. Bring that same energy in on the next inhale and let it spread from your forehead down your neck and shoulders. Allow it to permeate your chest, each arm and across your belly and lower back. Feel it releasing your legs and feet. Let it settle into you for a few minutes longer. All you need to do is breathe.

As you begin to bring your awareness back to the room, to your body, take a deep breath in and exhale it with an audible "aaah". Wiggle your fingers and toes, wrinkle your nose. Pull one knee up to your chest and then the other. Give yourself a hug and rock slightly from side to side. Notice your regular breathing. Is it full? Is it any different than at the beginning of today's practice?

*Shanti, shanti:* Peace. Namaste.

## PRACTICAL APPLICATIONS

• The rigidity and involuntary muscle contractions that come with Parkinson's and other movement disorders don't always respond to stretching. In fact, stretches can cause more tightening by triggering muscles into further contraction. Breathing can calm these muscles enough to let go of their grip.

• Breathing deeply helps increase circulation.

• Deepening your breath can clear your mind.

• Quieting breaths can also prepare us for sleep, which is especially useful with restlessness, a side effect that often accompanies medications for movement disorders.

• Depression is another symptom of disease or side effect of medications. The release of tension and lowering of stress hormones that result from deep breathing exercises can help alleviate the symptoms of mild depression.

## YOGA TO GO: APPLYING IT TO YOUR DAY

• Take note of your breathing pattern at least once a day. Is it shallow or deep, quick or slow?

• Next time you're waiting at the doctor's office, rather than leaf through a magazine, spend a few minutes becoming aware of your breath.

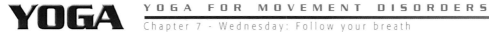

Try to deepen your inhales and exhales filling the belly and rib cage.

- Use the few moments at a red light to take a few full breaths.

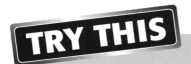

**A FOOTBALL TRICK**

During breathing exercises, or simply during the Coming to Stillness part of practice, if it's difficult to get air through the nose, as can happen especially with stroke, try this. Use the nasal strips that professional football players wear. The adhesive strips open up the airway for fuller breaths (which means more oxygen in the blood, which means more energy). The strips can be found at most drug stores and are easy to adhere. They even come in clear (and glasses can be worn over them).

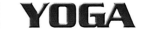

# Chapter 8
# THURSDAY: STAY STRONG

*'I do believe I'm feeling
stronger every day'.*
**– Feelin' Stronger Every Day, Chicago**

Callie's head injury occurred in the months between eighth grade and freshman year in high school. Through the summer, she never missed her twice-weekly physical therapy sessions. Her walking improved as she practiced on the treadmill and worked with weights and Thera-Bands. Her wit hadn't been affected and she smiled and joked easily.

As September closed in, she didn't chat and laugh as much. She said she'd rather keep coming to the clinic than go to school. There'd be kids there she didn't know and the ones she did know hadn't seen her all summer. Either way, she'd stand out limping down the halls with a dangling arm. Worse yet, the occupational therapist had shaved that arm. And her smile was crooked. She did not want to step foot into that high school.

It took as much emotional strength as it did physical strength for her to walk through the doors of that school. Not only did she go, she grinned as she told everyone at the clinic about her teachers, the drama club sign-ups, the cute boys. She frowned for a few seconds as she mentioned the cheerleading tryouts. She said she figured the coaches would say she wasn't strong enough yet. If they only knew....

## ASANA PRACTICE

Virabhadrasana, or warrior pose, builds strength and stamina in the face of battle, the everyday challenges as well as the life-changing ones. There are three warrior poses. In the first two, the reach is in opposite directions. The back arm and leg represent the past and the front limbs symbolize the future. While our hands and feet are reaching for both what was and what will be, our minds and bodies remain centered in the present moment. It's helpful to keep this in mind while in the poses, noticing if your body is leaning forward or back rather than balanced in the middle.

### Coming to stillness
Find a comfortable seated position on your chair or on a cushion on the mat. Press your sitting bones down as you lengthen up through the crown of your head. Inhale deeply through your nose, pause, and exhale.

On the next deep breath in, slowly count until your inhale is complete. Pause, and exhale to the same count.

On the next inhale, count again. On the exhale, let the count go two beats longer than the inhale. Count again, slowly, on the next inhale. Allow the exhale count to go four beats longer than inhale.

Return to your regular breath but notice if you're feeling anything different in any part of your body.

## Warm-ups
Please refer to Chapter three for the warm-up exercises to do before practicing the following asana flow. Work through all of Set A and 1, 4, and 6 from Set B.

## STRENGTH POSES
*Seated Warrior Flow*

*Need: Straight-backed chair*
*Sticky mat, Blocks (2)*
*Blanket (optional), Strap (optional)*

**Difficulty: Any level can try this set of poses.**

Set up your mat and chair so there is room for your legs on either side when you turn in your chair. Have your blocks handy.

1. **Warrior I:**

a.  Turn to the left and sit sideways on the edge of your chair. Place your left foot on the floor in front of you, knee bent at a right angle.

b. Set a block on either side of your left foot.

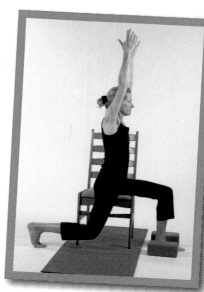

c. Kick your right foot back behind you, toes on the floor. Alternately, you can drop your right knee straight down from your hips to rest on the mat or a folded blanket.

d. Inhale and reach up with both arms, elbows straight, palms facing each other.

*Seated Warrior I*

2. **Forward bend:** Exhale, hinging at the hips, and place your hands on the blocks. Inhale up and return to center. Turn to the right and repeat Steps 1 and 2. Return to center.

3. Take a resting breath. Notice if you sense any changes in your arms and legs.

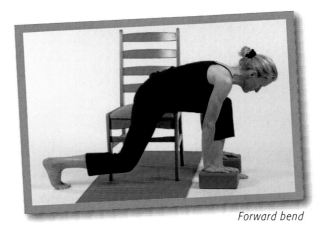

*Forward bend*

4. **Warrior II:** Step your legs wide, left leg bent at a right angle at the knee, right leg straight, foot flexed and heel on the floor. Pressing down into the left foot and out through the right heel, lengthen through the crown of your head. On an inhale, raise your arms to T position, your left arm parallel to your left knee. Relax your shoulders as you reach out through your fingertips. Gaze out over your left fingers.

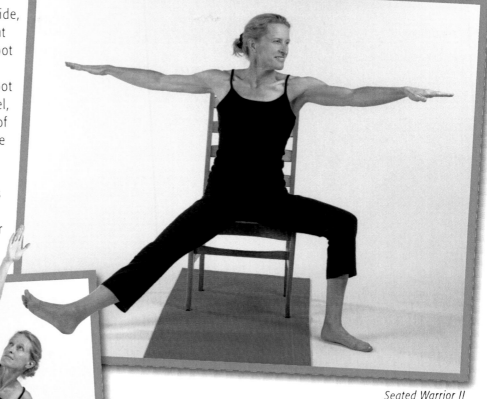

*Seated Warrior II*

5. **Wide angle:** Drop your left elbow to your left knee. On an inhale, sweep your right fingertips up, exhaling them over toward the left. Try to you're your elbow straight but not locked and your arm in line with your ear. If your neck feels comfortable, look up at your raised hand. Inhale back to center.

6. Repeat Steps 4 and 5 on the other side.

*Wide angle stretch*

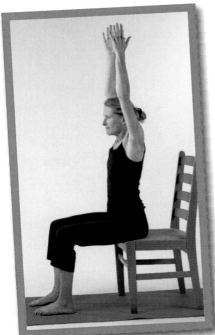

*Seated Warrior III*

7. Return to center and notice any sensations in your arms.

8. **Warrior III:** From seated mountain, inhale and raise both arms up, reaching through fingertips and the crown of your head. Exhale and hinge forward at the hips with a straight back as you lower your upper body and extended arms towards being parallel with the floor. Note that this is an upper back strengthener. If you feel any pain in your lower back, come out of the pose and take a resting breath.

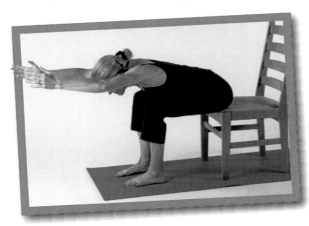

9. **Yoga mudra:** From warrior III, inhale and reach your arms behind your back, interlacing your fingertips. On an exhale, point your knuckles back and up toward the ceiling. Inhale. Exhale your palms to your knees, inhaling back to upright.

• If your hands don't reach each other, feel free to use a strap. Clasp the strap in each hand behind your back and point your hands back and up. Relax your arms and release the strap. Exhale your palms to your knees and inhale back to upright.

*Yoga mu◖*

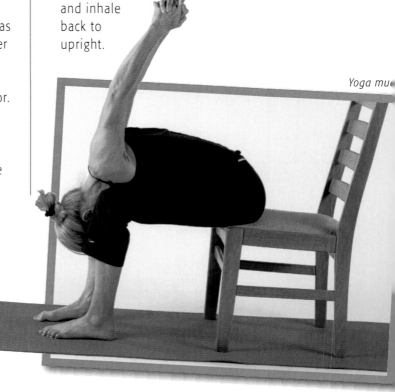

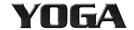
10. **Bicycle legs:** This is an abdominal strengthener. Place your hands behind your sitting bones on the back of the chair. Find your balance as you lift both legs, slowly pedaling an imaginary bicycle. Alternately, keep one foot on the floor as you lift the other leg toward you then away before switching feet.

11. Take a resting breath and prepare for the Relaxation that follows.

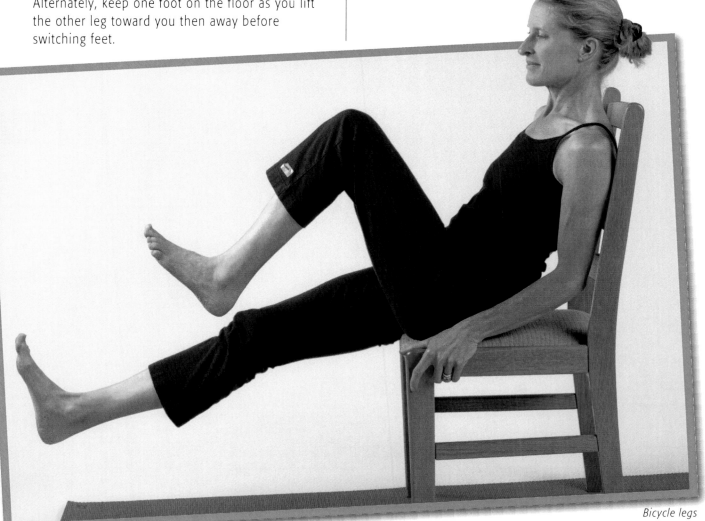

*Bicycle legs*

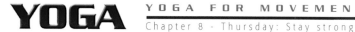

**STRENGTH POSES**
*Standing Warrior Flow with Tree*

*Needed: Two straight-backed chairs*
*Sticky mat*

This can be a challenging and energizing flow. If you have balance or overheating concerns or are new to stretching and strengthening, try the seated variation first.

Place one chair at the end of the mat, all four legs on the mat, with the back facing you. Have the other chair handy.

1. **Warrior I:** Stand in mountain pose and place your hands on the chair back for support.

    a. Step your right foot back, knee straight but not locked, and press down through the heel.

    b. Bend your front knee, making sure it is lined up above your ankle, not beyond it.

    c. With equal weight pressing down through the front and back legs, raise one or both arms, elbows straight and palms facing each other. If it is comfortable for you, look up at your hands.

    d. Alternately, keep both hands on the chair back for support and look forward or slightly up.

e. Step back into mountain pose and switch legs, stepping your left foot back to repeat on the other side.

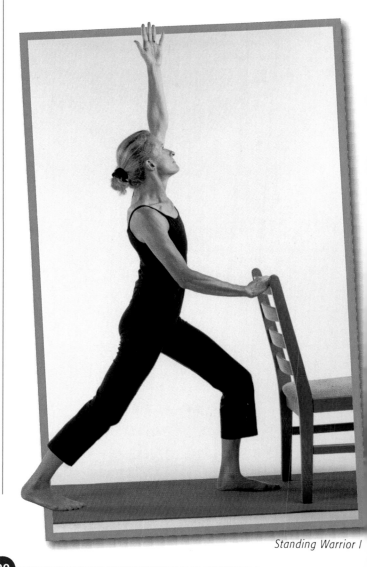

*Standing Warrior I*

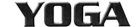

2. **Warrior II:** Stand in mountain pose and place your hands on the chair back for support.

   a. Step your right food back and pivot, turning sideways to the chair.

   b. Place your left foot so it is pointing at the chair. Position your right foot so the outside is parallel to the back, short end of the mat.

   c. Bend your left leg, making sure your knee is lined up above your ankle, not beyond it. Your right leg remains straight. If you can, press into the ball of the front foot and the outer edge of the back foot.

   d. With an inhale, raise your arms to a T position, your left arm parallel with your left thigh.

   e. Turn your gaze to look out over your left fingertips.

3. **Wide angle:** Drop your left hand to the chair for support. Inhale and raise your right arm up, exhaling it overhead. Inhale back to center and step your feet together into mountain pose. Take a resting breath.

4. Repeat steps 2 and 3 on the other side, with your right foot pointing at the chair.

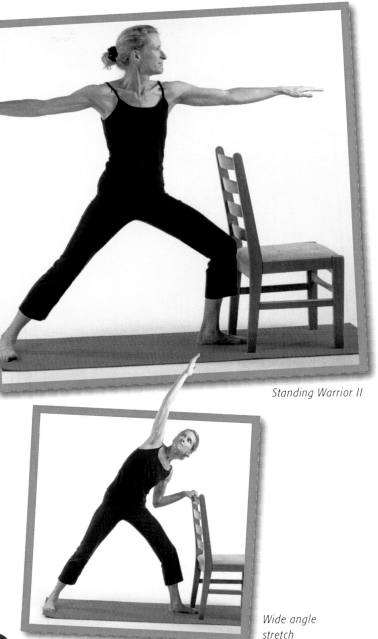

*Standing Warrior II*

*Wide angle stretch*

The next poses are for helping and increasing balance.

5. **Warrior III:** Face the back of the chair.

   a. From mountain pose, place your hands on the chair back and shift your weight to your left leg.

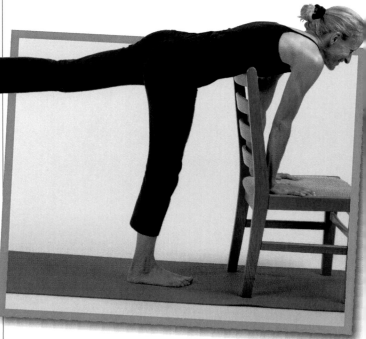

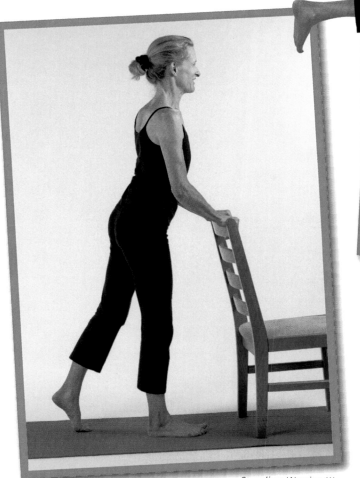

*Standing Warrior III*

   b. Inhale and step your right leg back, toes on the mat.

   c. Exhale as you hinge forward at the hips, raising your back leg as your torso lowers. Reposition your hands on the chair as needed for support.

   d. Inhale back to mountain pose.

6. Repeat Step 5 on the other leg.

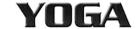

7. Position the second chair opposite the first with enough room between for you to stand between with outstretched arms. You should be able to touch the back of the chair with your fingertips for support.

8. **Opposite hand to knee:** Stand in mountain pose with a chair on either side of you. Raise your left knee and tap it with your right hand. Step the left foot down and raise your right knee and tap it with your left hand. Alternate between the two for four more rounds. Reach out to either chair as needed for support.

*Opposite hand to knee*

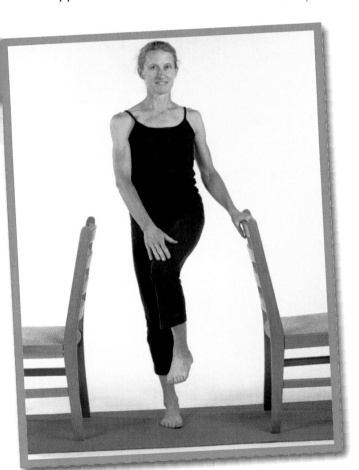

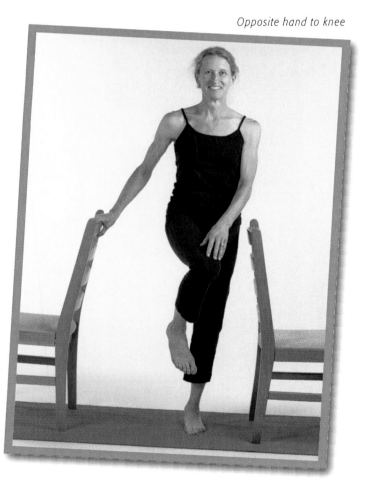

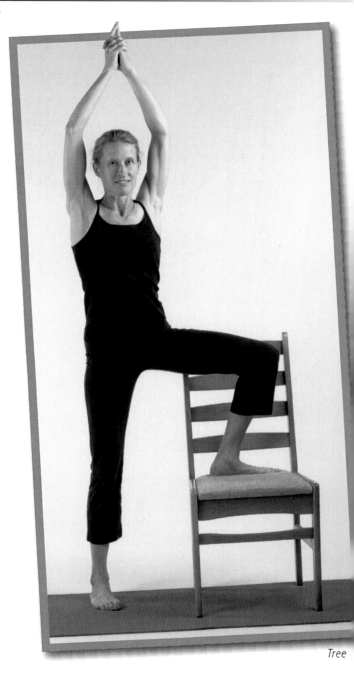

9. Turn one chair so the seat is facing forward. You may remove the second chair or keep it in place for added support.

10. **Tree:** Stand in mountain pose directly beside the chair.

    a. Shift your weight to the leg further from the chair.

    b. Using your hand on the chair back for support, place the leg nearest the chair on the seat, knee bent and at a right angle to your body. This stretches the inner thigh muscles.

    c. With your weight mostly on the straight leg, press down, rooting through your foot and extend up through the crown of your head and out the bent knee, like the tree trunk, strong yet flexible.

    d. If it feels comfortable, inhale as you raise your hands overhead, fingers interlaced, index fingers pointing up.

    e. If you can, balance in tree for thirty seconds before returning to mountain pose.

    f. Take a resting breath and move to the other side of the chair for tree pose on the other leg.

11. Shake out your limbs. Remove the chair from the mat and prepare for Relaxation.

*Tree*

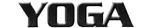
## RELAXATION: GUIDED IMAGERY

Lie in a comfortable position, cushioned and supported under your head and neck and warmed by blankets. Place a bolster under your knees to relieve any strain in the lower back Try an eye pillow (remove glasses or contact lenses first) if the room is bright.

Let yourself settle onto the mat. Feel the floor support the back of your head, shoulders, back, hips and sacrum, thighs, calves. Let them all be still, releasing into the mat, the floor, the earth.

Breathe and feel the air fill the back of your lungs, the back ribs expanding and contracting.

Allow your awareness to go to the back of your head, neck, shoulder blades. Breathe in to any tension in your upper back, down the spine to the small of your back down to the tailbone. Follow your breath down the backs of your legs, hamstrings, calves, and heels. Feel them pressed into the earth, letting go.

Notice the front of your body. Feel the air on your face. Let you brows, eyes, jaw go slack. Breathe peace into any tension in your chest and shoulders, arms and open palms, abdomen, hips, thighs, shins, toes.

Supported by the earth and open to the sky, you are in the balance between what is behind you and what is before you. Like a warrior, strong while relaxed and in balance. Rest this way for several more minutes.

As you begin to bring your awareness back into the room, into your body, wiggle your fingers and toes, wrinkle up your nose. Pull one knee into your chest and then the other. Roll to one side and rest there. Note the sensations on the back of your body, on the front. How are they similar or different? Slowly push yourself up to seated and let your eyes ease open.

May you be grounded yet free. Namaste.

## ESPECIALLY BENEFICIAL

• Getting up from a chair or out of bed is difficult when there's weakness on one or both sides. The warrior poses build strength in the arms and legs, which can ease the transition from sitting to standing.

• Fatigue is a common symptom of a number of movement disorders. Practicing strength and balance poses increases our stamina and can fend off fatigue.

• Balance work helps reduce falls and improves our posture.

## YOGA TO GO: APPLYING IT TO YOUR DAY

• If you can, try putting your socks on while standing. Lean on a wall or stand close to the edge of the bed for safety.

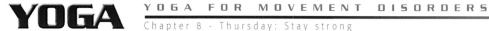

• Sit in front of a mirror. Notice if you're fully upright, shoulders even. If not, before correcting yourself, close your eyes and feel the position. Open your eyes and make any adjustments. Close your eyes again and sense any difference.

• The symptoms of stroke, Parkinson's, MS, and any number of movement disorders involve loss: loss of balance, muscle control, abilities. Rebuilding strength is important, but take a few moments during the day to consider the strengths you have: strength of character, a strong sense of design, a great listener and friend, an authority on roses or birds or jet engines.

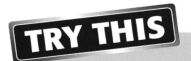

**TAKE FIVE**

Take five minutes. Take them for yourself. Take and sit with those five minutes each day in a favorite spot. Maybe include a favorite pillow. Sit together with those five minutes as you would a dear friend, quiet together because you need no words. Sit with each other, indulging in this special time daily. Those five minutes of simply breathing reset your body, refresh your mind, and restore the mind/body connection.

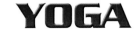

# Chapter 9
# FRIDAY: FLOW

*"Smooth runs the water where*
*the brook is deep".*
**– Henry VI, William Shakespeare**

Ruth dreaded swimming lessons as a child. Riding the school bus in the summer was bad enough. Add to that, the shouts and squeals echoing off the cinderblock walls, chlorine biting at her nose, the icy cold water – it all made her shiver.

Skinny and awkward, she barely floated and flailed about gasping for air while the other kids learned the crawl and the breast stroke. She hid her towel and declared it lost, hoping that would save her from having to continue. She lingered over her bowl of corn flakes in the morning figuring that if she missed the bus, she wouldn't have to show up at the pool.

Ruth did master the lessons from childhood, knew various kicks and what to do to stay afloat. But thirty years later, she said she decided it was time for more. She practiced twice a week for two months, stopping after each lap to adjust her arm movements or work on her kick. She knew she was getting stronger but said she felt mechanical.

Standing in the shallow end of a lane one day, she strapped on her goggles and decided to simply let the water support her as she moved in rhythm with her breathing. Gliding through the pool, she emerged again sixteen laps later. She'd learned how to swim.

## ASANA PRACTICE

So much energy goes into a pose, following the steps for which arm to stretch up, whether the elbow is straight or bent, aligning, grounding, reaching, and of course, breathing. Focusing on certain muscle groups at a time is good for isolating areas of tension or that need strengthening. Asana practice can also be fluid, flowing from one pose to the next. This can happen by stringing certain poses together that meld into one another. This also occurs when we stop trying so hard to do the pose and, instead, stay aware of our breath and let the pose happen.

With many movement disorders, motion is jerky, awkward, and stiff. Practicing yoga in a flow helps remind our muscles that they are fluid, that there is grace within.

### Coming to Stillness
This combination of a mantra, or repeated phrase, and mudra, or hand gesture, stimulates both sides of the

brain where the voice follows the breath and the finger movements flow with the voice.

As you recite each syllable of the mantra, one fingertip on each hand touches your thumb, each time creating a circle. The mantra itself is a circle, symbolizing the cycle of life. It is Sa Ta Na Ma and translates as Beginning, Life, Death, and Rebirth. Like the round form the fingers and thumb make, the pattern of repetition starts where it ends.

**The finger motion is**

**Sa** – index finger to thumb

**Ta** – middle finger to thumb

**Na** – ring finger to thumb

**Ma** – pinkie finger to thumb

Begin in seated mountain pose with your eyes closed. Rest your hands on your lap, palms up, index finger and thumb tips touching on each hand. Take a deep breath in. On an exhale, recite the mantra as your fingers flow with each syllable of it, reciting the mantra ten times as follows:

Two times aloud

Two times in a whisper

Two times silently

Two times in whisper

Two times aloud

When the cycle is complete, sit for a few moments, letting your breath settle back into its regular pattern. Notice any sensations in your fingertips, any vibration in your chest. Gently open your eyes and move to the warm-ups.

*Warm-ups*
Please refer to Chapter three for the warm-up exercises to do before practicing the following flow.

*Poses*
This flow ends where it begins, continuing the circle. Once the steps become familiar, try repeating the flow one or more times, keeping your movements fluid. Consider playing soft music, the same piece or pieces each time, while flowing through these poses. The music can help cue some of the movements.

**CIRCLE OF POSES**
*Seated Circular Flow*

*Needed: Straight-backed chair*
*Sticky mat*

**Difficulty: Any level can try this flow.**

Sit in mountain pose at the edge of your chair seat.

1. **Upward salute:** Inhale as you slowly raise both arms to the sky, palms facing upward. If it feels comfortable and you feel stable, have a look up at your hands. Turn your palms to face out and exhale your arms down.

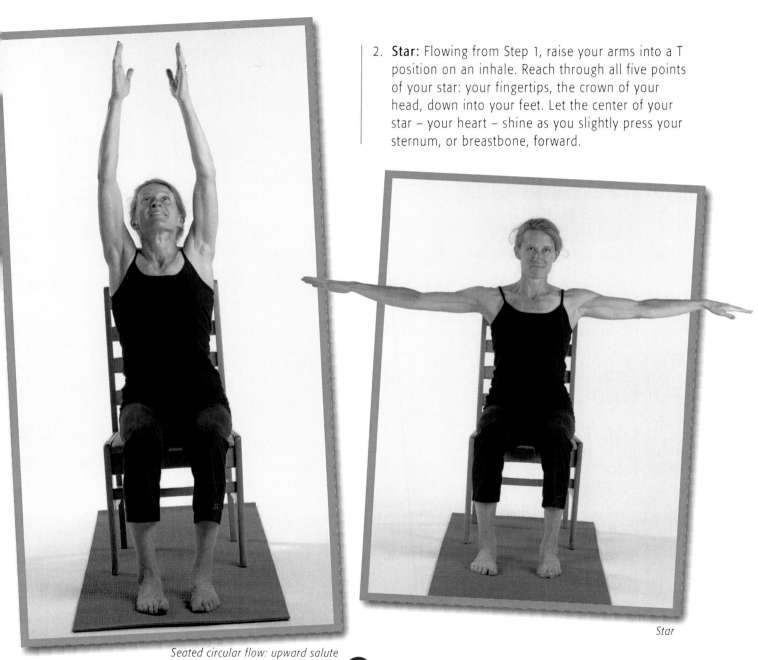

2. **Star:** Flowing from Step 1, raise your arms into a T position on an inhale. Reach through all five points of your star: your fingertips, the crown of your head, down into your feet. Let the center of your star – your heart – shine as you slightly press your sternum, or breastbone, forward.

*Seated circular flow: upward salute*

*Star*

3. **Stargazer:** Keeping your arms straight, inhale while you raise your right fingertips to the sky, your left to the ground.

Look up at your right fingertips. Exhale back to star and inhale your left fingertips to the sky.

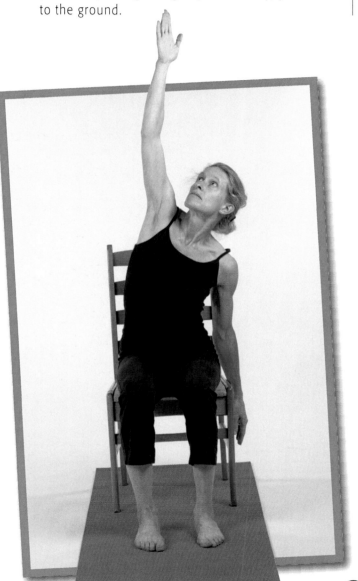

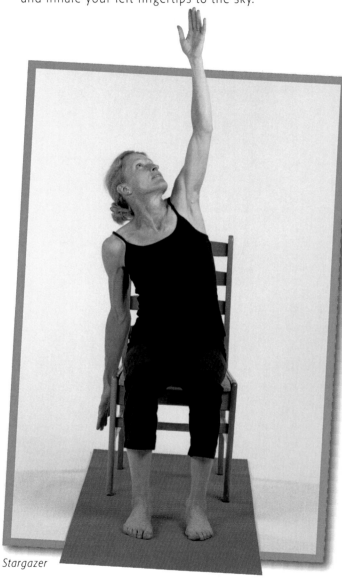

*Stargazer*

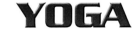

4. **Twist:** Inhale back to star. Bend your elbows and place your fingertips on your shoulders. Following your breath, inhale center and exhale and twist to one side; inhale center, exhale and twist to the other side. Repeat three times, ending on a twist to the right.

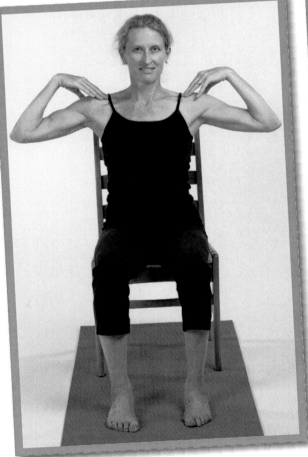

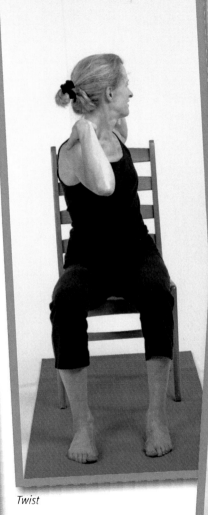

*Twist*

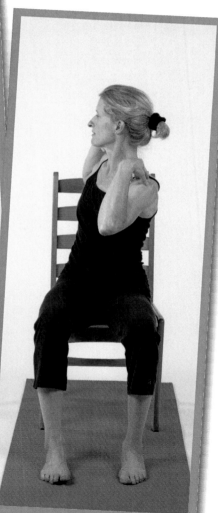

5. **Wide angle stretch:** Straighten your right arm and gaze out over your right fingertips. Inhale and raise your right arm straight overhead. Exhale as you bend your upper body, reaching your    fingers towards your left knee. On an inhale, straighten, and repeat the twist in Step 4 two more times, ending on the left. Repeat the wide angle stretch for the left arm.

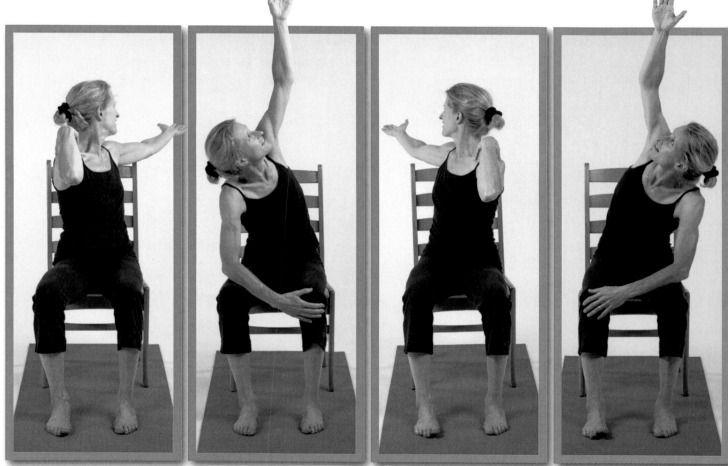

*Wide angle stretch*

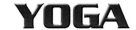
6. **Clasped-hands shoulder release:** Flowing from Step 5, straighten back to center, raising both arms overhead on an inhale, clasping your fingers together and turning palms up. Reach through your hands and crown of your head, keeping your shoulders relaxed. Exhale your arms in front of you, fingers still clasped but palms turned in to face you. Let your upper back round and drop your chin slightly, opening up the shoulder blades. Inhale as you release your clasp and bring your hands behind your back, once again clasping your fingers, palms facing your back. Exhale your elbows straight as you raise your sternum and gaze slightly.

- If your hands don't reach behind your back, use a strap. Clasp the strap behind your back where it is comfortable for your hands.

7. Release and inhale back to seated mountain pose.

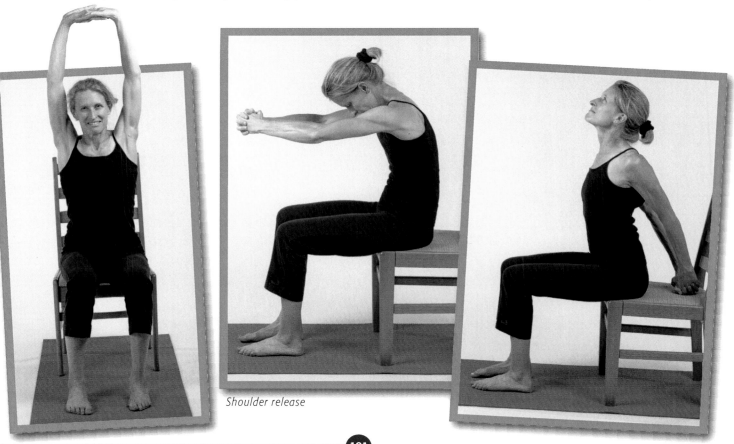

*Shoulder release*

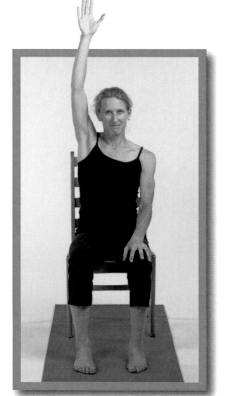

*Raised arms*

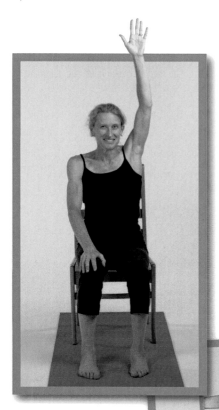

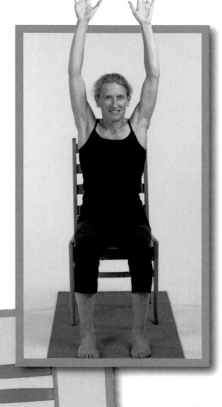

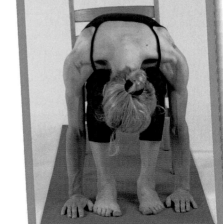

8. **Arms up:** Release your hands to your knees. Inhale and sweep your right hand overhead, exhaling your hand back to your knee. Inhale and sweep your left hand overhead, exhaling back to your knee. Inhale and sweep both hands overhead, exhaling into a forward bend, hinging from the hips with a straight back.

9. **Upward salute:** Inhale up, raising your arms to the sky, palms facing upward.

10. Exhale arms down, back to seated mountain, and take a resting breath before preparing for Relaxation that follows.

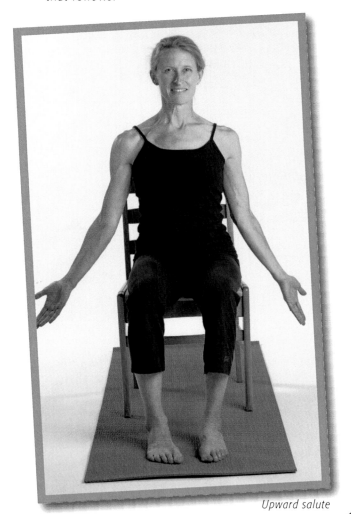

*Upward salute*

## RELAXATION: GUIDED IMAGERY

As you adjust to lying on your mat, feel the floor beneath you, solid. Let your whole body – your head, shoulders, back, legs – be fully supported and cushioned by blankets or a bolster. Inhale deeply through your nose, pause, and exhale it all out through your mouth.

Close your eyes and let them relax. Allow your jaw to soften, your forehead to be smooth. Imagine a mountain stream. Picture the stream at its beginning, at a waterfall high up in the rocks. Clean, clear water. Listen as it rushes between the rocks, splashing into a pool below. Watch as a droplet springs from the waterfall and dances and swirls in the stream that flows past roots and pebbles, through the countryside into a lake at the base of the mountain. On a warm day, the drop evaporates before it condenses again in a cloud that will send it back to the waterfall. Now watch as a droplet from the waterfall lands on the crown of your head. It flows through you, dancing and swirling into any space that needs fluidity. Let it wash into your lower back or across your knees, gliding in, clean and clear. Watch as the droplet reenters the stream that flows to the lake. Rest for a few more minutes, knowing that the cycle will continue and that you are fluid.

As you begin to bring your awareness back to the room, take several deep breaths. Wiggle your fingers and toes, wrinkle up your nose. Pull one knee up to your chest and then the other. Give yourself a hug and rock slightly from side to side. Before you sit up and open your eyes, notice if any part of you feels lighter, freer, more fluid.

May peace flow like a river within you. Namaste.

## ESPECIALLY BENEFICIAL

• Some movement disorders affect the strength of our voices. Like singing, chanting mantras increases our lung capacity and diaphragm control, both of which contribute to strong vocal projection.

• Rigidity and involuntary contractions can soften with gently, flowing movements.

• Attaching rhythmic movements to the regular beat of music can help with motor block, which is what happens when we get "stuck" or "frozen" in mid-step. Moving to music can help. Recalling the familiar beat of a song when "stuck" can help muscle memory associate the beat with movement.

## YOGA TO GO: APPLYING IT TO YOUR DAY

• Ask your doctor if swimming is right for you.

• Drink a glass of water. Taste it. Feel it on your tongue and as it goes down your throat.

• Notice your breath as you listen to water falling – raindrops, a shower, a melting icicle.

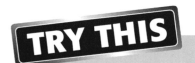

### GREEN RICE

Studies suggest that green tea's antioxidants may be helpful to people with Parkinson's because it protects dopamine neurons. Besides a cup or two in the morning, try leftover green tea in soups or in lieu of water when cooking grains (green tea with jasmine makes for flavorful rice).

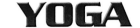
# Chapter 10
# SATURDAY: RESTORE

*'Renew thyself completely each day;*
*do it again, again, and forever again'.*
**– Chinese inscription cited by Thoreau in *Walden***

Before class begins, the studio is quiet as people ease into stretches or simply sit in their chairs, absorbed in the moment.

Enter Joe. A new student with a round, boyish face and an impish grin, he is talking to anyone and everyone. Laughing and chattering, he takes a seat. Sentences continue to crash into one another well into the warm-ups. His stroke has clearly not affected his speech.

We move through neck and shoulder rolls. Small pockets of stillness settle between his words. As we gently work through seated poses, there are longer pauses. I watch his shoulders drop, his fingers unfurl as he relaxes in the chair.

When it is time for an ending restorative pose, he lies back on the mat, a blanket rolled up under his knees, another folded for a pillow, a lighter one draped across him. He does not speak. He simply breathes.

The restorative power of a fully supported pose grounded him, released him from the nervousness that can throw any of us off balance and cause us to prattle

on too much or too fast. He later said he slept quite well that night. Now that's something to talk about.

## ASANA PRACTICE

Restorative poses differ from regular asanas. Rather than actively reaching and stretching, restorative poses passively allow opening to occur. The body rests in any of a number of positions propped by blankets, bolsters, rolled-up towels, pillows, weighted bags. Gravity and the deepening breath allow for release. Grounded by the earth solid beneath us, restoratives help renew the smallest cells and bring light to the darkest mood. No need to wait until the end of the week to enjoy these poses.

### Coming to stillness
Before finding a comfortable seated position, choose one of the following poses and set up your props for it. That way, you can move smoothly from a relaxed position into the few warm-ups and on to the restorative pose. These asanas are somewhat labor-intensive to set up, with lots of folding and positioning of props. But, they're well worth the effort once you've settled into the supported pose.

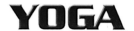 
Once you've arranged your blankets and blocks, find a comfortable, straight-backed position on a cushion, on the mat or in a chair, with your palms resting on your knees or with your hands on a pillow in your lap. If you're in a chair, position your hips at the rear of the chair seat so that your spine can rest on the back of the chair. If you're on a cushion or the mat, consider sitting so that your back is against a wall for added support.

Gently lengthen your spine by reaching up through the crown of your head while pressing down through your sitting bones.

Allow your eyes to close. Soften the muscles in your face: your brow, your jaw. Feel your body supported from below and from behind. Notice if you can feel your feet in contact with the floor, your sitting bones against the cushion or mat. Allow yourself to sink into the support, settling down and back.

Inhale deeply and pause your breath to the count of two. Let your exhale be an audible aah. Inhale and exhale this way two more times.

## Warm-ups

Working through a few warm-ups before a restorative pose opens up the spine and can help align joints. This provides for a deeper relaxation during the restorative pose. Rather than following the full routine of warm-ups, move through 7, 8, and 9 from Set A and 2 and 4 from Set B (please refer to Chapter three for the warm-up exercises).

## Poses

Three poses are listed here. Each has a different restorative benefit. Choose the one that best fits your needs at the moment. The first is a calming pose, the second refreshes, and the third pose is nurturing.

## SUPPORTED BASIC RELAXATION
*Floor variation*
*(Or, couch or bed variation)*

> *Need: Bolsters or sofa cushions*
> *Blankets and towels (up to 5)*
> *Sandbag or bag of rice (optional)*
> *Eye pillow (optional)*
> *Timer (optional)*

**Difficulty: Anyone can try all three of these poses.**

In this first position, bolsters and blankets support your body as you lie on your back. This is an overall calming pose that can help slow your heart rate and quiet the central nervous system.

The floor's solidity provides better support for this pose, but if getting down onto the floor is difficult, this position can be done on a couch or in bed.

Set up the resting – or what I like to refer to as nesting – space by spreading a blanket, folded in two length-wise, on the floor for cushioning. Place small towels or washcloths folded once on either side of the blanket, about mid-way down. These will support your wrists.

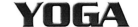
If your legs need added support, have two sandbags or sacks of rice ready near the foot of your blanket. These can be placed at the outside of your legs, along the knees and shins, to keep your legs from rolling out too much.

Have a bolster or sofa cushion handy to place under your knees.

Fold another blanket or towel for your head and neck. Be sure that the folds provide enough support so that your chin points directly toward the ceiling, not tilting back or tucked forward. If you'd like, have an eye pillow or washcloth folded lengthwise handy for lightly covering your eyes (remove glasses or contacts first).

You may want to set a timer. If you do, try to use one that has a peaceful sound rather than a jarring one so that you're not jolted out of your relaxed state.

Finally, have another blanket ready for covering up against cold. It is important not to get chilled because it will become too difficult to relax. Also, with Parkinson's and with MS, body temperature regulation gets off kilter and once the body gets cold, it can take some time to get warm again.

Once the props are in place, consider using the bolster to sit on for Coming to Stillness so that it is a smooth transition to this restorative pose.

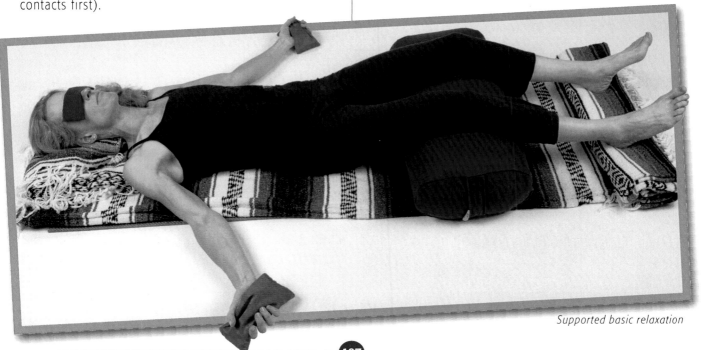

*Supported basic relaxation*

1. After the three rounds of breath in Coming to Stillness, slide off the bolster down to the blanket. Arrange the bolster under your knees and the sandbags or sacks of rice, if you're using them, beside your legs.

2. Place your wrist supports in position so that you can reach them once you've reclined.

3. Use a blanket to cover yourself to keep warm if the room is at all cool.

4. Lie back and rest your head on the folded towel or blanket and place the eye pillow or folded washcloth over your eyes to block the light. Rest your wrists on the small folded towels or washcloths.

5. Breathe. Inhale and pause as you did in Coming to Stillness. Exhale with an audible *ahh*. Let your entire body – bones, tissue, organs – all settle into the supports. Smile. Feel that smile travel to your bones, tissue, organs.

6. Breathe your normal breath and relax in this pose for at least fifteen minutes. Twenty would be okay, too. So would thirty.

7. To ease out of the pose, keep your eyes closed as you wiggle your fingers and toes. Remove the eye pillow and scrunch up your nose.

8. Take a deep breath in and out. Pull one knee to your chest. Push the bolster away slightly with your other leg before pulling that knee to your chest, hugging both knees in. Roll to one side and rest there for a moment.

9. Pressing your hands into the floor, push yourself up and sit for a moment. Notice your breath and the sounds around you. Bring your awareness to your body, to the ease that has settled in, even a little. When you're ready, open your eyes and rejoin the world.

## INVERTED RESTORATIVE POSE
*Elevated Legs*

*Need: Blankets (2)*
*Chair or sofa or bed*
*Sandbag or sack of rice (optional)*
*Eye pillow (optional), Timer (optional)*

In Elevated Legs pose, the feet are positioned higher than the heart, inverting blood flow. This can reduce swelling in the ankles and help with restless, involuntary movements in the leg muscles. It can be used to refresh after overdoing. Please note: anyone with glaucoma or high blood pressure should check with a doctor before practicing this pose. Also, if you have a head cold or sinus infection, avoid this pose until you've recovered.

Set up for this pose by spreading a blanket, folded in two length-wise, on the floor for cushioning. Place a straight-backed chair on one end of the blanket, or, spread the blanket perpendicular to the edge of a sofa or bed.

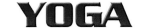

Place one small towel or washcloth, folded once, on either side of the blanket, about a foot from the chair, sofa, or bed. These will support your wrists. Have another blanket handy if needed to cover up to stay warm. If you're using a timer, have that handy as well.

Fold another blanket or towel for your head and neck. Be sure that the folds provide enough support so that your chin points directly toward the ceiling, not tilting back or tucked forward. If you'd like, have an eye pillow or washcloth folded lengthwise handy for lightly covering your eyes (remove glasses or contacts first).

Once the props are in place, consider using the chair (or sofa or bed) to sit on for Coming to Stillness so that it is a smooth transition to this restorative pose.

1. After the three rounds of breath in Coming to Stillness, gently come off the chair and lie down on the blanket on your back, facing the chair. Swing your legs up onto the seat of the chair, knees bent and calves comfortably supported.

2. If you're using a sandbag, place it across your shins. This helps keep your legs stable, allowing your hips and thighs to completely let go of doing any of the work keeping your legs in place.

3. Adjust the blanket under your head and neck for comfort and chin alignment.

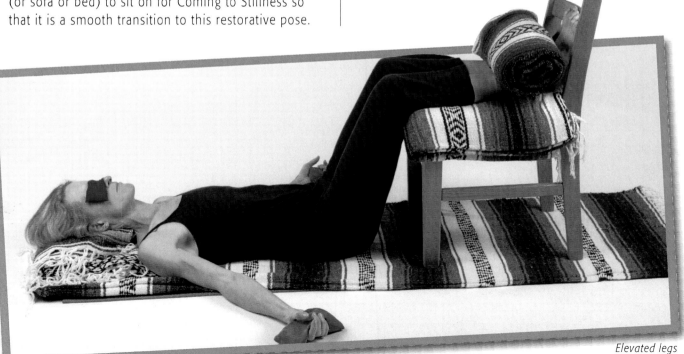

*Elevated legs*

4. Place your wrist supports in position so that you can reach them once you've reclined.

5. Use a blanket to cover yourself to keep warm if the room is at all cool.

6. Lie back and rest your head on the folded towel or blanket and place the eye pillow or folded washcloth over your eyes to block the light. Rest your wrists on the small folded towels or washcloths.

7. Breathe. Inhale and pause as you did in Coming to Stillness. Exhale with an audible ahh.  Let your entire body – bones, tissue, organs – all settle into the supports. Smile. Feel that smile travel to your bones, tissue, organs.

8. Breathe your normal breath and relax in this pose for ten to fifteen minutes. Twenty would be okay, too. Come out of the pose if your toes begin to tingle from lack of blood.

9. To ease out of the pose, keep your eyes closed and wiggle your fingers and toes. Remove the eye pillow and scrunch up your nose.

10. Take a deep breath in and out. Wriggle your legs out from under the sandbag if you're using one. Pull one knee to your chest and then the other, hugging both knees in. Roll to one side and rest there for a moment.

11. Pressing your hands into the floor, push yourself up and sit for a moment. Give your circulation a chance to readjust. Notice your breath. Bring your awareness to your body, to any spark of new energy. With a smile, you're your eyes and continue living your day.

## SEATED RESTORATIVE POSE
*Child's Pose in a Chair*

*Need: Two straight-backed chairs*
*Sticky mat, Bolster or sofa cushion*
*Block or book(s), Blankets or towels*

This restorative pose is akin to a grown-up's version of a Time Out. It can reset your mood and bring you back into balance. It also opens up the back muscles while cradling the heart and mind.

To set up for this pose, place two chairs eight to ten inches apart, seats facing each other. Turn one chair slightly so a corner of the seat is facing the other chair. Both chairs should have all four legs on the mat to prevent slippage.

Place a block or books on the back of the seat of the chair that is not turned. Place the bolster or sofa cushion beside the chairs.

Fold the blanket or towel to fit the length of the bolster. If it is a long blanket, fold the end several times to form a pillow for supporting your head on the bolster. If the blanket is not long enough, fold a towel for your head to rest on.

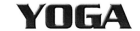

Have an extra two blankets or blocks handy if your feet do not rest comfortably on the floor when seated in the chair. Have your timer within reach, if you are using one.

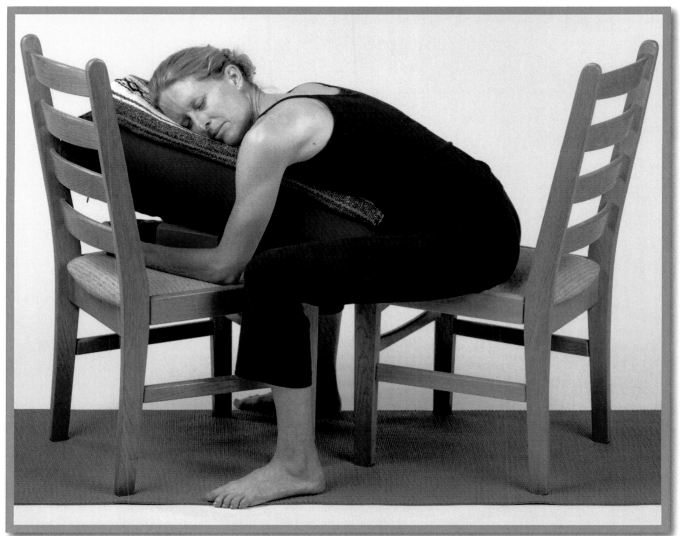

*Child's pose with chairs*

For a smooth transition to this restorative pose, consider using the chair that is turned to sit on for Coming to Stillness. Sit so that one of your legs is on each side of the corner of the seat that points to the other chair.

1. After the three rounds of breath in Coming to Stillness, reach for the bolster. Place one end on the corner of the chair you're sitting on and the other end on the block or books on the other chair.

2. Position the blanket and or towels on the bolster for your head support.

3. Check the position of your legs. Your knees and ankles should each be at right angles. If your legs are short, place a block or blanket or pillow under your feet until you get the correct angle of ankle and knee.

4. Bend forward to rest your belly and chest on the bolster, turning your head to rest on a cheek, and looping your arms under the bolster between the block and where it is resting on the seat of the chair. Let your shoulders droop and relax. Notice if there is any discomfort and rearrange props as needed.

5. Breathe. Inhale and pause as you did in Coming to Stillness. Exhale with an audible *ahh*. Let your entire body – bones, tissue, organs – all settle onto the supports. Close your eyes and let everything go quiet, all the chatter in your mind fall silent. Feel that stillness travel to your bones, tissue, organs.

6. Breathe your normal breath and relax in this pose for ten to fifteen minutes. Halfway through, turn your head to rest on the other cheek.

7. To ease out of the pose, keep your eyes closed and wiggle your fingers and toes. Scrunch up your nose.

8. Take a deep breath in and out. Stretch your arms out in front of you or to the sides.

9. Pressing your hands into the bolster, push yourself up and sit for a moment. Notice your first thought. Smile at it. Bring your awareness to your body, to any place that has settled into ease. Your Time Out is over. Open your eyes and enjoy your time back in your day.

## ESPECIALLY BENEFICIAL

• Relaxation is a key component of boosting the immune system and allowing for healing. Living with a movement disorder does not grant us a Get Out of Jail Free card for other illnesses or diseases. We still catch colds. Through relaxation techniques, such as regularly practicing restorative poses, you help your body stay strong.

• A fully relaxed mind and body will aid in both falling asleep and staying asleep for longer periods. This is particularly helpful for the insomnia often attached to Parkinson's or from side effects of movement disorder medications.

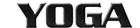

- Releasing tension throughout the body can ease tremor and involuntary muscle contractions.

- The rejuvenation that can come with the Elevated Legs pose can be a welcome bit of energy when fatigued.

- Restfulness in the face of stress is just plain good for ourselves and everyone around us.

## YOGA TO GO: APPLYING IT TO YOUR DAY

- If you drive, de-stress your car time. Drive at the speed limit. On the highway, let other cars pass with the same detachment, as if leaves were blowing by. Give yourself a few minutes extra to enjoy the ride.

- Create a morning ritual that is calming. Before getting out of bed, close your eyes and listen to your breathing. How quiet can you make it? Follow the sound inside. Notice any sensations in your body – cool air on your skin, an ache. Without judgment, breathe into those spaces. Smile.

- Take a moment in the beginning of your day to pause. Choose a place to sit for a couple of minutes – in your kitchen, outside in the yard, on a step – and close your eyes. When you open them, make note of the first color you see. Think of something that color that is soothing. Notice how many times you see that color during the day.

- Breathe. Notice when your breath is short or shallow. Treat yourself to a deep inhale and equally or longer deep exhale, at the grocery store, folding laundry, while working on the computer.

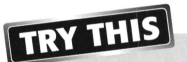

### TAKE CARE

Get a pedicure. Or at least soak your feet, massage them, rub lotion into the rough spots. With movement disorders, we sometimes forget about our feet. There are so many muscles and joints throughout the body to orchestrate simply to walk or climb a flight of stairs that our feet get left out in the cold. Or, always hidden away in socks. In yoga, we're grounded by our feet, even in many seated positions. Although the sensations aren't what they once were, there is still blood flowing into our toes, a set of nerves on our soles, a pulse at our ankles. Let energy flow between you and the ground. Expose your toes. Go barefoot. Feel the earth under your feet.

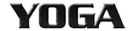 
# Chapter 11
# MEDITATION AND MORE

'Yoga is a light, which once lit,
will never dim. The better your
practice, the brighter the flame [4]'.
— B. K. S. Iyengar

Peggy Cappy closed her Yoga for the Rest of Us teacher training with a question: **What do you need to do next for yourself on your yoga journey?**

**I knew my answer immediately:** Add meditation to my practice. I recognized its many benefits. Meditation calms the mind, increases our capacity to cope, strengthens the immune system, opens new pathways in the brain. Still, each night, after I brushed my teeth, I'd mutter to myself in the mirror, "Oops, forgot to meditate today."

**My New Year's resolution:** Meditate. I added *meditate* to my to-do list, put sticky notes on my computer screen, bought a cushion - purple and soft - and set candles on my dresser. But at the end of the day, I'd be saying, "Oh, right, I was supposed to meditate."

## BEGINNING YOUR PRACTICE

One early morning when I awoke to a quiet house, I swung my legs over the side of the bed, wrapped myself in a quilt, and followed my breath in and out.

When the song lyric that had plagued me for two days started repeating itself, I focused on my breath. Thoughts swam in. *Don't forget to call about the gutters. Bring a salad to Beth's tonight.* I didn't wave them away or get annoyed. Instead, I recognized them as thoughts and brought myself back to the air moving in and out with each breath. A tremor crept into my thumb, settled in my wrist. I breathed into it.

When I opened my eyes, I stretched my arms out and glanced at the clock. Ten minutes had gone by. I'd done it; I'd meditated. Had I experienced an awakening? No. Though I did wonder about what my thoughts said about me and my state of being. *Gutters? Salad?*

But that's one of the points about meditation. We are not our thoughts—thankfully, or I'd be pretty dull given what pops into my head. Past events or conversations replay in our minds. Or, if you're more of a planner, future events or conversations preview in your head. In either case, we really have no control. How many times have I wished something would stay as it was, or expected an outcome and

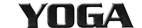

was disappointed when it didn't happen as I'd hoped? Coming back to the breath brings us back to the present moment, because the present moment is all that we truly have.

In meditation, we step back into a witness role and watch those thoughts of past and future, let them come and go without getting caught up in them. Simply notice them and gently return awareness to the breath.

### When and where

When we think of yoga we typically envision moving our bodies into various poses. The original yogis of the past, however, meditated. They developed asana practice years later to stretch before or between sittings so they could meditate for longer periods. Meditation came first.

Deciding where to add a meditation period – before or after or even at a separate time from your asana practice – is a personal choice. Early morning has the advantage that it may be the quietest time with least distractions. On the other hand, my muscles are eager to go with the first light of day and I find it easier to sit after I've moved around for an hour or so.

The length of time and number of times a day or per week that you meditate is different for each of us. Starting with ten minutes a few times a week is a good beginning. Expand the length or number of days as you feel comfortable. Or, if you tend to get

overly stiff from not moving, try sitting for ten minutes several times during the day rather than sitting for an hour at a time.

### Props

You can sit or lie down for meditation, though, often, when I lie down I fall asleep. I find that sitting on a straight-backed chair is best for comfort, though I do sit on the edge of the bed at times. A pillow in your lap makes a good support for resting your arms. If your legs are short, use a folded blanket or firm pillow under your feet to bring your legs to a position where there are right angles at the ankles, knees, and hips. Keep another blanket handy in case you feel chilled while sitting.

The keys to staying alert are to maintain a straight spine and to be comfortable. Even with the softest pillows and the best intentions, though, the mind has a tendency to wander. Stephen Cope, a psychotherapist and senior Kripalu yoga teacher, likens sitting for meditation as tying a puppy to a post [5]. Our puppy minds are active; they especially object and tug at their collars when we tie them up and say, Stay. But, eventually, our endless thoughts, like the puppy, will lie down and relax.

### TECHNIQUES

There are numerous styles, approaches to, and venues for meditation. If you're interested in learning more, yoga studios, various churches, and continuing education courses offer classes. Group meditation guided by an instructor can be a helpful way of staying focused.

If you're distracted by someone coughing or breathing deeply, you may prefer sitting solo. There are audio CDs available that lead you through meditation steps and visualizations. Choose what works best for you.

Listed here are only a few of the many meditation techniques.

## IN AND OUT

*Needed: A straight-backed chair or cushion*
*Blanket or pillow (optional)*

This technique is one that I come back to again and again for its simplicity. It uses the breath as the focal point. Once you are in a comfortable, seated position, close your eyes or let the lids drift partway closed. Inhale a full, slow breath through the nose and say to yourself, "In." As you exhale through the nose, slowly and fully, say to yourself, "Out."

Thich Nhat Hanh, a Vietnamese monk, Zen master, and author adds to this [6]. After several rounds of breath, inhale a full, slow breath through the nose and say to yourself, "In. Relax." And, on the exhale, say to yourself, "Out. Smile."

To end your session, sit for another moment and notice if anything feels different, lighter or heavier, warmer or cooler. Slowly open your eyes. Smile.

## OBJECT

*Needed: A straight-backed chair or cushion*
*Blanket or pillow (optional)*

This technique uses a visual to focus on during the meditation. The object can be a candle, a vase of flowers, a postcard of a place you've been, a photo of someone you love, a seashell. Once you're in a comfortable, seated position, gaze at the object for several breaths. Next, gently close your eyes and keep the image in your mind. Continue your slow, steady breathing as you picture the object. If your mind wanders or you need a reminder of what the object's details are, open your eyes part way and glance at the object before closing your eyes again.

To end your session, sit for another moment and notice how your body feels. Mentally scan from your head to your toes. Is your jaw relaxed, your brows not furrowed? Does your back feel ready to bend and move? Are there any other sensations you notice?

## VISUALIZATION

*Needed: A straight-backed chair or cushion*
*Blanket or pillow (optional)*

For this technique, you use your imagination to envision relaxation and healing. Once you're in a comfortable, seated position, As you breathe, focus on a particular ache or area of your body. Picture the ache or sore area as a new bud, still tightly closed. Imagine

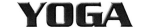
the warmth of the sun on the bud and picture it gently opening into a flower. Or, use another image of something taut that you'd like loosened, such as a gnarled fist into a smooth open palm, a butterfly emerging from a cocoon, snow melting and evaporating.

To end your session, sit for another moment with the open image in your mind – the flower in full bloom, for example. Really let yourself see it so you can recall that soft, smooth image any time during the day.

## ESPECIALLY BENEFICIAL

• The visualization technique helps break up the knots that build up from involuntary muscle contractions.

• As meditation practice becomes a part of your day, like brushing your teeth, you'll find you don't want to skip a session. A daily practice relaxes us in mind and body on a regular basis, keeping stress levels down.

• Your constant companion is you. Meditation lets you tap into that essence and be with it without judgment.

## MEDITATION-TO-GO: APPLYING IT TO YOUR DAY

• The In, Out technique is available at any time of day. Try it for a few breaths at the dinner table, in the shower, at the corner store.

• There is plenty to explore to deepen your knowledge of yoga and meditation: classes, books, DVDs. They cover material from an in-depth study of the breath to the essence of yoga to the history, variations on poses and the limbs of yoga.

My fears and worries don't disappear during meditation. They still exist, but the calm that comes with a session allows me to step back, bring the fears and worries into balance. It's like rearranging the letters in an anagram, making one word or phrase from the same letters as another. The tiger is always there. But I've reordered its hold on me. It's no coincidence that *meditation* is an anagram of no, *I tamed it*.

Whatever it is that you want to tame, wherever you choose to go with yoga and meditation, be gentle, breathe, and enjoy your journey.

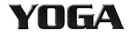

# References

1. Cappy, P. (2008) Interview with Lorie Parch, Yoga Journal, "Forever Young." August, p. 135.

2. Folan, L. (2005) Yoga Gets Better with Age. Emmaus, PA: Rodale Press.

3. Hackney ME, Kantorovich S, Levin R, Earhart GM. Effects of tango on functional mobility in Parkinson's disease: A Preliminary Study. Journal of Neurological Physical Therapy, Vol. 31, December 2007.

4. Iyengar, B. K. S. (2008) Yoga, The Path to Holistic Health. London: D K Publishing.

5. Cope, S. (2006) The Wisdom of Yoga: A Seeker's Guide to Extraordinary Living. New York, NY: Bantam.

6. Hanh, T. (1991) Peace Is Every Step: The Path of Mindfulness in Everyday Life. New York, NY: Bantam.

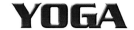

# Bibliography

Cappy, P. (2006) *Yoga for All of Us: A Modified Series of Traditional Poses for Any Age and Ability.* New York, NY: St. Martin's Press.

Christensen, A. (1999) *The American Yoga Association's Easy Does It Yoga.* New York, NY: Fireside.

Cope, S. (2006) *The Wisdom of Yoga: A Seeker's Guide to Extraordinary Living.* New York, NY: Bantam.

Devi, N. (2000). *The Healing Path of Yoga: Alleviate Stress, Open Your Heart, and Enrich Your Life.* New York: Three Rivers Press.

Farhi, D. (2003) *Bringing Yoga to Life: The Everyday Practice of Enlightened Living.* New York, NY: Harper Collins.

------ (2000) *Yoga Mind, Body & Spirit: A Return to Wholeness.* New York, NY: Henry Holt and Company.

Folan, L. (2005) *Yoga Gets Better with Age.* Emmaus, PA: Rodale Press.

Hanh, T. (1991) *Peace Is Every Step: The Path of Mindfulness in Everyday Life.* New York, NY: Bantam.

Iyengar, B. K. S. (2008) *Yoga, The Path to Holistic Health.* London: D K Publishing.

Kraftsow, G. (1999) *Yoga for Wellness: Healing with the Timeless Teachings of Viniyoga:* New York, NY: Penguin Group.

Lasater, J. (2003) *30 Essential Yoga Poses: For Beginning Students and Their Teachers.* Berkeley, CA: Rodmell Press.

------ (1995) *Relax & Renew: Yoga for Stressful Times.* Berkeley, CA: Rodmell Press.

Long, R. (2006) *The Key Muscles of Hatha Yoga.* Plattsburgh, NY: BandaYoga.

McCall, T. (2007) *Yoga as Medicine: The Yogic Prescription for Health and Healing.* New York, NY: Bantam Books.

Sacks, O. (2007) *Musicophilia: Tales of Music and the Brain.* New York, NY: Knopf.